MEND TH

*A transformative journey
from deep despair
to spiritual awakening*

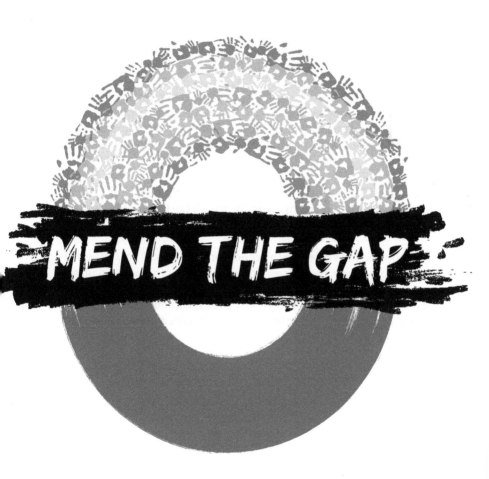

MEND THE GAP

KATIE MOTTRAM

RƎTHINK PRESS

First published in Great Britain 2014
by Rethink Press (www.rethinkpress.com)

© Copyright Katie Mottram

For Mum, so that you can finally emerge from the chrysalis
that has held you dormant for so many years,
and be the butterfly you were born to be.

PRAISE FOR MEND THE GAP

Reading the profound insight that Katie Mottram shares within these pages stirred my soul like rainfall on parched land. Finally, someone was speaking to my questioning heart with such familiarity. Deep emotions began to flow and personal desire to play a part in the mental healthcare system transformation was re-ignited. It felt as though Katie knew my mind and shared the very same path. I believe Holy Spirit brought this book of powerful perception and visionary Katie Mottram into my life for a Divine purpose. Katie's incredible passion and heart of gold has contributed to the paradigm shift of mental health services like a key going into the ignition of a "vehicle of change". One in which I'm delighted to be alive to witness and also climb aboard. The mental health care system won't be able to ignore the pearls of wisdom throughout this book.

A copy of *Mend the Gap* needs to be given to every student entering the field of psychiatry, along with anyone practising in the field or experiencing a personal crisis. It's time to put Soul back into the treatment of spiritual beings having a human experience. The word 'Psyche' is ancient Greek for 'Soul'. With books of awareness like *Mend the Gap*, I feel hopeful that a holistic approach to mental health treatment will no longer be 'Greek' to the profession of psychiatry.

Rev. Laurie J. Nevin
Ministerial Counsellor (www.lifenavigator.ca)

AUTHOR'S NOTE

This book is completely based on factual events in my life. Individuals and organisations are called by their real names, except where pseudonyms have been used to protect the identity of some individuals. I would like to thank each and every one who has played a part in my journey, without whom I would not be where I am today. We are all unique, and yet interconnected beyond logical belief.

My aim is that, by being so open and frank, *Mend the Gap* will support those who are working to transform the mental health care system, and provide proof that those changes to acknowledge the transformative power of dialogue are most definitely needed. I also pray that it gives hope to those who may be suffering right now, that there really can be light at the end of the tunnel. I hope that it enables people to be brave and more outspoken about their own experiences and emotional turmoil; that these can be owned and normalised, and that those who hear the stories can be more open-minded about how experiences can be interpreted. It is my ultimate aim that *Mend the Gap* will act as a building block in the bridge that "mends the gap" between spiritual experience and psychiatry.

CONTENTS

FOREWORD

Reading and experiencing Katie's memoir, a story from her life, has been humbling and touching whilst also immensely inspiring. Although this memoir reminds me of the common criticisms of mental health services, I am surprisingly sanguine about the future of those services. But we have a long way to go. As a lead clinician in one of the many mental health services that are engaged in a recovery model, I consciously attend to 'mini-memoirs' every day. The model purposively encourages the telling of 'mini-memoirs' or recovery stories which are similarly humbling and sometimes distressing whilst inspiring and touching. Thankfully, they are also perpetuating and constructing a sign of hope that such 'memoirs' will be heard and recognised as a new paradigm of understanding that mental distress is for many a completely natural phenomenon and part of a transformative human process.

But we need to be brave if we are to move onwards. There have been and are many brave clinicians, professionals and peers who, like Katie, have spoken up and spoken out about their concerns for and about traditional services. I am one. I, like Katie, have struggled for many years to accept that mental distress is anything other than that which the individual understands it to be. As professionals, we may believe we have the answer in a treatment or a therapy. We worry about cause and effect, about costs and standards. We pathologise, we diagnose and prognose – all potentially iatrogenically harmful for many. We focus on clinical recovery but that clinical recovery can lead to a 'career' in mental health services – more potential iatrogenic harm. And I believe we have missed a trick, in that the answer is there: it is within the individual who suffers the distress. The cause and effect is within, rendering the cost to be low and the standard high. To be with a person to help them look within, to make sense of what has happened when, for a time, it may make no sense at all, costs little but is of the highest quality of care. I have personally intuitively believed that as one human being helping another, the most useful human being I can be to another in mental distress is one that truly listens; truly believes that the distress is an individual experience that can be best explained by the person experiencing it; and in that, the experience is what the individual understands it as. This may have made me unpopular and 'soft and woolly' and 'a pushover' with no 'evidence-base' – not 'clinically sound' with my colleagues, but proportionately as popular with my real peers, those peers known as my 'patients'.

The missing trick is also hidden within personal recovery, rather than clinical recovery. Katie has given us two wonderful examples of how, with help, both she and her mother have made sense of their distress and what had happened, about how they could recover from that distress and how they can learn about it and about themselves along the way of their own personal recovery journeys. Katie has taken us one step further in her memoir within her explanation of her understanding of her distress, and in her description of her spiritual crisis she has helped us step further up on the bridge of understanding between the mental health world and the spiritual world. Katie has been brave to tell us this memoir, this story of her life; we need to hear more brave stories and we need to be brave and listen and believe and recognise how much of the person's story is vital to a personal recovery journey.

It is widely acknowledged that most mental health services are currently organised to meet the goal of clinical recovery. But how then do we transform services towards a focus on personal recovery? I believe the seeds to this transformation have been sown; the recovery journey of services has started; the first tide is turning; the forums are out there; and many, many professional are comfortable, willing and able to engage in the concept of shared expertise – to understand the part they play in the recovery relationship and the value of the understanding of the lived experience. These professionals have been brave and need their organisations and commissioners of services to also be brave. To bravely recognise that the costs and quality are hidden within personal journeys rather than clinical journeys.

Similarly, the understanding of spirituality in mental health is augmenting but there is no point in us exploring, explaining and understanding the wider sense of spirituality, if we don't understand it fully, to its widest extent, to the extent of many lived experiences, memoirs and recovery stories. If we don't do this we will have missed a trick: a very simple trick; a very simple truth. This truth is out there; we just need to hear it, open more discussions about it and, as professionals, we need to look within ourselves, understand our own spirituality and allow it to guide our own recovery journeys before we can embark on a recovery journey with our peers. This is how as a nurse I can enhance my skill into a craft, an art form.

So we need to be brave, we will need to take some risks if we are to do things differently, if we are to make the required paradigm shift that will move us from a service which focuses on professional expertise to one that responds to 'human need'. We need to mend that gap...

> *'Only those who will risk going too far can possibly know how far one can go.'*
>
> T.S. ELLIOT

Sue Howlett, Registered Mental Health Nurse and Recovery Project Lead.

INTRODUCTION

We all have a story to tell, and although mine may be different to yours, there will be themes of "being human" that unite us. It is in owning our stories and accepting ourselves as we are, that we are able to let down barriers, embrace our true selves; in so doing we become connected and also the best we can be as individuals.

I'd always known intuitively, since being a young child, that there was more to life than I was being told, that society was missing something that must be pretty crucial in some way – *surely this mundane experience wasn't all life was about*? I had spent a depressed adolescence and an avoidant early adulthood, battling to understand, searching for answers (to what question I wasn't really sure). This futile search had only resulted in a heavy sense of having to pretend to be someone who "fitted in" with the material, secular, mechanical world that we still see today, because that was all I knew about surviving the twists and turns of life.

It is hard to believe that, having worked in the mental health system for over fourteen years, I had never heard the term "spiritual emergency" until it happened to me! I had kind of "drifted" into this field of work, desperate to understand my own mum's mental struggles after she had been diagnosed with an ever-changing cacophony of debilitating labels when she tried to commit suicide and then say that she believed she was a "healer". Her beliefs completely disregarded, my poor mum was sectioned, medicated and given brutal electro-convulsive treatment, rendering her an almost robotic existence. Mum was told she was mad, and so that was what she was forced to believe. It didn't sit right with me somehow, but all of the "professionals" were saying it, and I was scared of her behaviour, so it must be true. I think I had reasoned that by gaining as much knowledge as I could about mental illness, it would protect me from going down the same rocky road. I now know that no amount of formulated learning can prevent us from experiencing a natural truth when our soul is ready, even if that truth is one that is not yet acknowledged within mainstream society and our Ego fights to believe it. I now know how wonderful and frightening such an experience can be, especially when nobody believes you, and how brave you have to be to believe in the experience for yourself, and listen to the message contained within it.

> "...one day, some great opportunity stands before
> you and calls you to stand up for some great
> principle, some great issue, some great cause. And
> you refuse to do it because you are afraid....
>
> Well, you may go on and live until you are ninety, but...
> the cessation of breathing in your life is but the belated
> announcement of an earlier death of the spirit."
>
> MARTIN LUTHER KING

I am thirty-eight, and I am afraid about speaking my truth, but I am more afraid of the consequences of not speaking it at all. Now my soul is alive, it refuses to go back to sleep. I discovered what I was searching for, and it was truly worth the wait and even all of the pain.

In this book I lay myself bare, documenting significant, sometimes traumatic, life events that I believe played a part in shaking my consciousness enough to learn the valuable life lessons needed to live life to my full potential and discover my soul's purpose. A purpose I would never have dreamed possible had somebody other than the Universe told it to me. In *Mend the Gap*, it is my very personal aim to relay (what I consider to be) some vital information about mental distress that isn't openly acknowledged in current Western culture. The opinions I express throughout the book are based upon my personal experiences; they are solely my own and are not intended to reflect the viewpoints of any of the professional bodies, to which I am connected. Much of the information is channelled from spirit but has been filtered by my human brain, which can be biased and still has much to learn! Otherwise it is information I have sought or come across over the last couple of years living and researching my spiritual journey. The information I am relaying is intended to make the reader think; it is not intended to be prescriptive, but rather to act as a tool, with which to open minds and encourage self-exploration. My desire is to de-jargonize the often complicated language that is used in this field, and to help create a bridge between the psychiatric establishment and spiritual world in order to create a new paradigm of understanding, that mental distress is something that can be a completely natural phenomenon, and part of a positive transformative process.

I've written this book from a distinctly specific, perhaps unique, position; the daughter of someone who has had the great misfortune to have spent half of her life being labelled, sectioned, and treated as "mentally ill" by conventional medicine and, paradoxically, as a mental healthcare worker, employed within the very field that, essentially, almost destroyed my family. On a profoundly intimate level, I've both witnessed and experienced the ill-making, often "deadening" effects of what happens when the soul remains largely ignored. It is my sincere hope that this antiquated system will evolve significantly within both my mum's and my lifetime. It's taken me many years to mend the gap within me; but, ultimately, I've used this once-blurry lens of experiential and philosophical duality to sharpen a dormant, yet persistent sense of purpose – one I would never have dreamt possible had the Universe itself not revealed it to me during a profoundly spiritual experience; a true spiritual emergency in every sense, that was impossible for me to ignore.

It is my sincere hope that, through revealing such raw and vulnerable moments and discussing the "universal truths" I believe they contain, you may find the courage to manage the spiritual and emotional hurdles of your own life...to dare to trust in and pursue your wildest dreams, regardless of challenges and set-backs, and to live within the fullness of your life's potential, unencumbered by fear or regret. Whatever your current life's circumstances may be, rest assured that you have access to a truly miraculous life; we are no different after all.

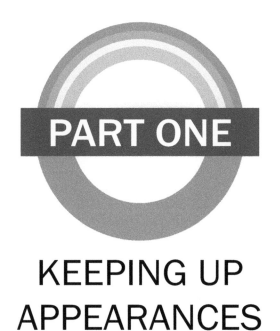

PART ONE

KEEPING UP
APPEARANCES

ONE

IT'S A MAD WORLD

*"Your brain tells you you've lost the plot,
but the little voice in your head tells you it
makes the most sense you've ever heard."*

Sitting beside her bed on the floor I had managed to get her to open up to me. I instinctively knew that by being physically lower than her I was reducing the amount of threat she must feel purely by the fact that I was staff and she was a patient. This wasn't text book stuff; it was natural empathy and human connection. I had learned enough through my own childhood experiences about how important it was to feel safe and listened to, as opposed to disempowered and controlled as a result of other people's insecurities. Her emotional scars were evident, not only visibly represented by the carvings all over her uncovered arms, but through her haunted eyes and the shakiness of her voice as she spoke to me;

"So what made you want to do this work then, surely there are better things to do than have to spend hours watching over the likes of losers like me?"

At least asking about me was giving her a reprieve from her own destructive thoughts for a short time. *But what should I say?* It was unprofessional of me to tell her any personal information, although it would be the truth and I didn't want to lie; she had encountered enough of that in her chaotic life. It wasn't surprising that it had been that, which had made her so distrusting of most people here.

My mind quickly drifted back to our first meeting just a few weeks earlier. Relatively new, at twenty-two, to the psychiatric nursing team, I'd been granted the "learning opportunity" of watching this equally young patient receive a course of Electro Convulsive Therapy for her recurrent, unresponsive depression. When I joined the staff in her room, they were already preparing to restrain and sedate her, earlier than necessary, just in case she tried to refuse treatment and became "uncooperative". *After all, how dare she try to resist their professional opinion on a treatment that was for her own good?*

Immediately, I felt uncomfortable being there – especially given my own mum's sordid history with such gruelling treatment – but my presence was clearly mandatory. If I wanted to work in the field of psychiatry, I must witness this brutal electrical invasion of this poor girl's brain. The plastic gum shield was placed between her teeth, a protection to prevent her from biting off her tongue whilst her body writhed in involuntary fits. I looked into her petrified eyes and, instantly, her face morphed into that of my mum. My heart raced and my head swam. I needed air. Without stopping to ask for permission, I stumbled my way to the door, my body desperate for natural light and a fresh breeze. Sitting on the concrete step outside brought a familiar sense of relief, for that brief moment nothing was real and I knew my own mind. Granted, I didn't know the scientific reasoning behind the use of electric current on the brain, but I did know that what I had just witnessed was beyond my own comprehension of "care".

Returning back to the ward I apologised for my moment of weakness, laughing it off as me being too squeamish. It was pointless me doing the full Psychiatric Nurse training if I was going to almost faint every time a painful procedure or disquieting moment arose. My nagging sense of worthlessness eating away at me, I wondered how I could ever make a difference in this field if I couldn't be stronger. Somewhere, deep down, I knew I had something to offer – but nobody could know about the flashbacks. No one could know I'd seen my mum's face unmistakably depicted in that moment of reflected pain. Otherwise, my colleagues would view me no differently than the patients I wanted to support. Otherwise, they may want to lock me up too. My silent tears must be confined to behind the locked door of the staff toilet. I must be strong.

When she was young this poor young woman had put her trust in the ones who were supposed to have been in charge of her care, the ones who were supposed to have loved her. But they had abused her trust. Why should she trust anyone ever again?

As I sat beside her she searched my face for answers... for a glimpse of the truth she desperately longed to hear. *Losers like me*; the words, along with the patient's obvious feelings of self-loathing hung as starkly in the room as the fluorescent light fixtures above us. She wasn't aware that her own defensiveness was now her biggest obstacle, pushing most people from ever experiencing the gift of knowing her. But I, for one, could see beyond that defensive façade into the eyes of her beautiful, albeit broken, soul. I could read her fear and longing as if such feelings were my own. Ever-so-slowly, with each of us revealing just a little more about each other, I could see her inch past her pain in search of the hope that lay just beyond it.

And so, with this glimmer of hope in mind, I dared to tell her a little more about myself... that I had grown up with a mum who had long suffered with "severe and enduring" mental health difficulties, and that I had started to work in the field, I supposed, as a way of trying to gain a better understanding. I told her that it was very hard to see my mum on medication with horribly debilitating side effects; the kind that made her nearly robotic and unable to enjoy her life. I told my patient that I thought she was very brave to be able to talk about her struggles, and that I only wished my mum could be so open and forthcoming about her own, internal struggle. "Do you think that, maybe, you can start to find a better way to deal with your pain? Something that isn't so self-destructive?" I finally asked. Again, she searched my eyes, looking for the seed of trust she so desperately needed. I offered it in the most genuine smile I could muster, and she nodded, ever-so-slightly. It was all I could do to keep from jumping up and hugging her; but instead, I kept still and let the space between us fill with mutual acceptance and trust. In that rare and beautiful moment, we both knew a true connection had been made, created through the simple act of non-judgemental listening.

"What do you think you're doing down there?" The ward sister shot me a disapproving glare as she stuck her head through the solitary room door.

Connecting on a human level. Giving someone trust who otherwise has none. Being an equal and genuinely interested, rather than acting like I'm on patrol. That was what I wanted to say. But, of course I didn't. Instead, like a guilt-ridden, reprimanded teenager, I quickly sprang to my feet, and sat back on the chair guarding the door, mumbling a string of apologies and half-hearted excuses to a senior colleague who'd already moved on to another room. *What did I know?* I'd only been in the mental health game "officially" for a year or so; I clearly needed more strict professional boundaries. As soon as the ward sister walked back into the corridor, my "observation subject" made a deft grab for a plastic tape cover to snap, creating a sharp edge which she quickly pierced into her already mutilated skin. I quickly wrestled the makeshift knife away from her; but, the connection severed between us loomed much larger and more painfully than any minor flesh wound. All the progress my young patient had made by finally allowing a sliver of trust and hope to enter had evaporated in that single, shame-creating instant. Officially the "enemy" again, I knew I had deeply failed her. I should have spoken out and refused to move. A look of vacancy filled her eyes as the nursing staff rushed in, pushing past me to deal with the commotion. I could do nothing but walk away, seething with anger: Who had the bigger problem here, I wondered; a young lady who was unable to control the depth of her emotions, or an older "professional" parading a veneer of self-control under a façade of power? I knew with whom I felt most comfortable, with whom I truly empathized – and that, in itself, frightened me. Yet, on the other hand, I also didn't want to end up bitter and so numb I appeared as heartless as many of the staff managing the psychiatric wards I had experienced. It felt like a no-win situation.

Hours later, at home after my shift, I remained bitter, angry, frustrated, and helpless to managing the undeniable "gap" between what I intuitively knew was right and what was being taught and expected of me. After going for a long run, propelled by more energy than usual due to the surge of emotion I felt inside, I opened a bottle of wine. How could no one else see that the incident today arose from feelings of powerlessness... from reducing an already distrusting, vulnerable young woman to feeling like even more of a burden to everyone, including herself? Surely, it wasn't bloody rocket science, was it? I poured my anger into a long letter of complaint, and then proceeded to rip it up. I knew that the way the system was currently being run, it wasn't helping people. Things needed to change – but how? And, how could I continue to be part of a system in which patients were treated so disrespectfully, that they weren't allowed to have even the smallest voice in their own care?

Maybe it would help release my pain if I cut my own arm? No, I knew it wouldn't; but, I certainly understood the motivation. *It sure was fucking painful keeping all this shit inside.*

Amazingly, by the time I started my next shift, I'd managed to compartmentalize my feelings enough to carry on as "normal". I convinced myself that I was young, naïve, and in need of more experience. Certainly, nobody would take my point of view seriously until I'd proven myself; so that would be exactly what I would do!

Despite nobody saying anything, I knew that I wasn't the only one amongst my colleagues who went home and drowned their sorrows in a few glasses of wine, or an episode of a miserable soap opera, in order to make their own lives feel more bearable. *Wasn't that the norm?* When things become a bit unmanageable it's okay to just distract yourself from reality for a while by getting drunk, eating crap, going on a holiday, spending money on things you can't afford to get a buzz, even dabbling in a few recreational drugs – *after all, everyone does it don't they so what's the problem?* Except I didn't want to join in the escapism as I knew deep down that was all it was. I wanted to understand, but the more I tried to resist, the more alienated I felt. *What was wrong*

with me? I was even failing at playing the game. *Why wasn't anyone admitting that they too felt insecure when I could blatantly see people falling apart all around me?* The people you least expected, the seemingly strong ones, were ending up on the other side of the "sanity" fence. Obviously falling apart was a weakness, and something I needed to hide. Just as my mum had needed to do, I became numb to emotion, to enable me to cope with my disillusionment and confusion.

There were similarities between some of the things, about which my clients confided in me during my successive jobs in various mental health roles, and what my mum had said when she had been sectioned years previously. Some, like her, had been deeply emotional and sensitive, afraid of what they were saying but desperate to be heard in some way. Some talked about "feeling strange energies", "being guided by a light", "communicating with spirits" or having extra special information from God. My training had taught me that these were signs of psychosis, of something going wrong within the brain (although nobody quite seemed to know what, exactly) that needed treating, pathologising and controlling back to "normality". These people were clearly bonkers and not just a little bit unsettled inside. Thank goodness I knew the score and could distance myself with the proper, professional lingo. *How on earth had I ended up working in this stressful mess?* I wondered...

TWO

UNDER THE SURFACE

She held me in her arms and looked into my eyes. I was supposed to have been her answer to everything... the missing puzzle piece that would finally fill the void. Yet, nothing – not even her indescribable sense of love for a new born baby totally reliant upon her – seemed able to overcome the profound longing for deeper meaning she'd wrestled with since childhood. In fact, in many ways, my arrival only pronounced such longing all the more.

Mum had always intuitively known that there was more to life than she'd been told; that modern society, as a whole, had a universal habit of overlooking a fundamentally deeper sense of purpose and meaning. As a result, she'd spent a depressed adolescence and an avoidant early adulthood battling to understand the chasm of unspoken yearnings within, as if in constant search for answers to questions she had never quite been able to articulate. At the same time, she was desperate to "fit in" to the materialistic, secular, mechanical world in which she lived, and tirelessly looked to find ways to conform, to mould herself into being something that she wasn't – someone who didn't spend countless, quiet hours searching for the meaning of life, but

21

rather lived contentedly within its most superficial, modern-day constructs, which in actuality left her feeling empty and frustrated.

It is not surprising that she'd followed conventional expectations; it was the usual thing to do for someone so sensitive, unassertive and confused about life. From the day her dad had died, she had resolved to keep her questioning and sadness only for the family dog, Jill. Jill wouldn't judge her or tell her she was being silly or not old enough to understand. How was her caring family to know that by being protected from attending her beloved dad's funeral, it would be the very thing that would haunt her throughout her adult years, finally breaking her to smithereens? Surely existential questioning was beyond the concern of such a quiet and unassuming ten-year-old? Nobody was to know what was going on in the mind of a young tomboy, seemingly enjoying the frivolities of life, too busy jumping off roofs and playing outside to be affected by their protective whispers in the night. She didn't want to be a problem, and so said nothing about how she really felt.

Sitting at the top of the staircase she had listened to them making funeral plans. Waiting intentionally until she had gone to bed so as not to upset her with all the morbid and practical talk, they were doing the best they could to shelter her from any emotional harm. Tears streaming down her cheeks she concluded that they mustn't consider her of importance; why else would they be hiding such a big event from her delicate ears? Her dad had gone, and she needed closure. But she couldn't possibly cause any more problems on top of everything else, her mum and older sister already had enough to contend with. She must keep her worries to herself; with Jill to confide in she would be just fine. She knew at least the family dog understood her.

And so life went on, with her unexploded emotional bombs becoming more deeply buried under the practicalities of everyday life. Mum struggled increasingly with feelings of profound loss over the ensuing years, hiding from her own grief and incomprehension about death. She had resolved herself to be strong for her family, whom she loved dearly, keeping her woes to herself was the only option, she felt it would be too selfish to admit that she wasn't coping. It had been years since she had lost her dad, surely she should feel okay by now? Why was it still playing on her mind and the painful memories still seeping into her emotions? Time was supposed to be a healer after all.

To keep herself emotionally afloat, Mum tried desperately to go along with the frivolities of life that seemed to keep everyone but her happy. She'd dress in the latest fashions and attend dances at the iconic dance hall in the local town. That was where she met the man who would later become my dad. A smiley, seemingly happy-go-lucky young man, he threw a rescue raft out to Mum, and off they both sailed, into the proverbial sunset. With Dad at the helm, Mum could be a stowaway, no longer having to steer her own course, with a life of wife and mother clearly mapped out before her. Surely that would give her answers, a sense of contentment in what life was all about? Now she would have a life, on which to focus, and be able to put any questions about death well and truly behind her. But the emotional grenades weighed heavily, and they weren't going to just disappear.

Despite her happy marriage, Mum's life-long questioning quickly crept back in, haunting her internal monologue with a vengeance in the quiet moments of her days: *What is the meaning of life? Is there really a God? Why do bad things happen to good people? What happens after death? Am I alone or am I connected to something bigger in the Universe? Are these things I sense really real?* Unfortunately, any potential answers to Mum's deeply spiritual questions seemed to have been buried alongside her own father, himself a Methodist minister, all those years ago. It wasn't long before Mum's effortless smile was once again slowly replaced by a "lost", faraway look that spoke volumes to the state of her deeply unsettled mind and heart.

Mum wasn't the only member of the family who often seemed to exist somewhere "beyond herself". Nan, my mum's own mother, had the same vacant look in her eyes, and yet she always seemed content, in a distant kind of way. After my parents were married, she'd often join them for Sunday lunch, happily singing along to Songs of Praise later in the evening, lost in her own, private world. Nan and Mum seemed to have an unspoken connection that way, if only because neither of them dared to utter a word about their mutual awareness and interest in the spiritual realm. They did, however, quietly share a love for anything and everything related to the paranormal, frequently exchanging (but never discussing) books by the psychic medium Doris Stokes. Doris was a famous clairaudient of the time whose public performances and prolific media career had made her a household name in Britain. Having come from an era in which anyone who believed in this sort of stuff could have been accused of being a witch or given a lobotomy, Nan never spoke openly about her views. And so Mum inadvertently learned that she couldn't discuss her beliefs, or experiences, either. This unspoken "knowing" between them couldn't be an issue if it wasn't acknowledged, and so it became a covert interest for both women, their inability to speak about it isolating them further.

The Sunday evening telly blared out until it made Dad's ears bleed with words that made no sense to him at all. What a load of religious codswallop!

"There's a call comes ringing o'er the restless wave,
Send the light! Send the light!
There are souls to rescue, there are souls to save,
Send the light! Send the light!"

Nan smiled her toothless smile and her eyes shone with a contentment that caused even Dad to be inquisitive. Mum and Nan exchanged a glance, the love and understanding between them, at a level so deep that their human brains couldn't comprehend, hung in the air like a magical energy. Dad felt himself distanced by their connection, he didn't understand this weird stuff and all he could do was build more walls to protect himself from feeling frightened by it.

Mum's relief at feeling somehow understood for that brief moment was shattered by Dad's defensive response:

"*Antiques Roadshow* is on the other side."

He reached for the remote and felt the uncomfortable fear subside as he deflected his attention onto how much the fake Rembrandt would fetch at auction.

It stood to reason because of his giving nature that, most nights, my dad's best-laid plans for his own leisure time seldom passed without interruption; he was always going off to help someone with a plumbing problem, no matter how much it obviously pained him and caused him to grumble behind-the-scenes.

"I'll be right there. No problem!" would be his common, cheery reply to customers. In trying to please everyone else all of the time, Dad's willingness to disappear at the drop-of-a-hat triggered Mum's sense of unimportance, although she never told him as much.

Once a fabulous football player, Dad also had starry-eyed dreams of becoming a singer. Now, as a plumber trying to make a modest success of his own, inherited family business, the only people to hear his dulcet tunes were the neighbours whilst he took a shower. *Who was he to believe that dreams could come true?*

They all sat around and focused on the distraction of the TV in the background. The Antiques Roadshow had ended and given way to another episode of a depressing soap opera that nobody really wanted to watch, and yet nobody dared rock the proverbial boat by switching over again. The family depicted in the box on the corner shelf screamed and shouted at each other. The mother cried as she told her daughter how angry she was that she'd seen her nicking money from her purse for drugs, and told her to pack her bags and get out.

Dad shook his head. Did people really behave like that?

"I can't believe people actually talk to each other like that. Why can't people just learn to keep their feelings to themselves and not hurt one another?"

Weighing in at five pounds, fifteen ounces, I proved to be a small but rather demanding force of nature, arriving within less than four hours of the onset of labour, the trauma of which caused my mum to tear badly enough to require stitching. Initially, she tried to breast feed, but I had difficulties latching on and she had no choice but to give up. A colicky baby who cried relentlessly during those first few weeks of life, I possessed the power to make my mother's heart simultaneously burst with love and pride, whilst paradoxically fill with desperation and frustration. She felt she had failed – both in her inability to soothe me properly and to shake the dark, inner void she'd expected (and desperately hoped) my arrival would immediately vanquish. Unable to sleep due to my constant wailing, she began to superficially self-harm by scratching nervously at her arms, which caused a strange, red rash to suddenly appear. When she could think of no other way to calm either of our nerves, she would finally give up and retreat to her "safe place"; a section located at the bottom of the staircase. There, she would curl up and wait out my deafening wails until I'd finally cried myself to sleep.

Had she only realised that what was to come would turn out to be the very thing that helped me to find a sense of meaning in our lives, she may not have acted the way she did; but then where would we be now if she hadn't? *Am I actually grateful that my mum tried to kill herself?* With hindsight, these things seem that they were meant to be – but hindsight sometimes takes years to comprehend.

Whatever made mum think the answer was in a box of slug pellets nobody will ever know. *Well she probably wasn't really thinking at all was she?* Her logical mind overwhelmed by thoughts of hopelessness and shame; years of buried emotional grenades finally surfacing for the pin to be pulled.

So the doctors whipped her away from me and tried every which way to detonate those repressed emotions; "What was this all about, what on earth was a woman like her thinking to do such a thing when she had such a loving family around her?" They told her she must be mentally ill, it made no sense at all to their prying, professional but still judgemental eyes, unable to get her to say what was wrong, because she herself had no idea. The professionals who chose to focus only outwards through their narrow-viewed *DSM (The Diagnostic and Statistical Manual of Mental Disorders)* binoculars, so as to avoid having to look inwards at their own sense of hopelessness and confusion at life. Hiding behind their own professional facades, along with reams of intellectual jargon, helped them from having to admit they really had no idea about how to help this poor woman.

With one desperate act, poor mum had solidified an official label of "madness" from the medical community;, the kind that would require, (according to her psychiatric doctors), a lifetime of heavy medication, all of which were accompanied by horrendous side effects that prevented users from ever experiencing a true depth of emotion, even the ones most longed-for, such as happiness and joy.

On the surface, the potent cocktail of anti-psychotic medication Mum received seemed to provide a helpful reprieve from her inner turmoil. Yet, she now resumed her dutiful tasks robotically, functioning on a virtually emotionless plane, while simultaneously trying to prove that she was worthy of being a wife and mother. Knowing she had hurt him deeply, she now felt less deserving of dad's attention than ever. At the same time, Dad worked hard to repress his own sense of helplessness and fear, rather than express his anger and grief at the situation. He too felt like a miserable failure. Was he really such a bad husband that he made his wife want to kill herself? More emotional grenades formed within their layers of unspoken hurt, creating a potentially fatal minefield through which I tiptoed as I grew up, always waiting, intuitively knowing, that another explosion was only a matter of time.

THREE

THE GLIMMER OF HOPE IN TRUTH

I was dreaming again. It had been recurring for as long as I could remember. I was climbing a dark, steep, spiral staircase, leading to where, I wasn't really sure. All I knew was that behind the door at the very top, on which I tentatively knocked each time, was a mystical character who never wanted to answer.

Now, at the age of seventeen, I was suddenly reminded of that old dream as I approached my headmistress's house. I knocked on the door with the same trepidation I had felt in my dream; this was her territory, and although not unkind, she had a reputation for being extremely stern with her students. Even a few minutes tardiness could unleash a wrath few could endure without tears, which was quite ironic really, as the wearing of watches at school was banned. I took a deep breath, knowing the reason I'd been summoned here was far more significant than lateness. I had missed the French language exchange – an entire week's stay with a family in France – and, now at such a disadvantage compared to my fellow students, I was petrified that I would fail my exams. I imagined my headmistress looking severely over the top of her brass-rimmed spectacles, judging, condemning, and asking me pointedly what excuse I could possibly offer which had prevented me from making such an important trip. I would surely now fail my A-Levels; then what would I do? Without qualifications, I couldn't land a good job, or find a good husband, which, ultimately, meant that I'd never experience the secure, contented life I so badly coveted. The shit had really hit the fan, and it was all my doing. I suddenly wished this scenario would end like that old dream, and I would wake to find myself in my childhood bedroom, full of wonder and relief.

When the reception I received was, instead, warm and sympathetic, I thought at first that I must have entered the wrong house. My headmistress offered me time and understanding, accompanied by sweet tea; and in return, I slowly told her what had happened while I gripped the cup with clammy, shaking hands. What would my friends have thought if they could see me now, so unravelled and unsure of myself? I was always so concerned with what everyone else thought, much like my mum. I felt I had to closely monitor every little thing I said and did, in order to make sure it was "appropriate". It was an exhausting way to live, and I rarely felt I measured up. Now, as I sat shakily with this virtual stranger who could ruin my future in one fell swoop, I felt the arduous, inner duality of watching myself with disapproval as another part of me simultaneously grappled to find just the right words.

The trouble was there weren't any "right" words for the surreal events that had just occurred. And so, sitting at her kitchen table, I battled to push aside my insecurities, ignored the nagging internal voice that told me she would consider me "pathetic", and recounted it all as best I could:

"It was Tuesday morning, exactly one week before my driving test ..."

She put her hand up, as if to stop me. Gently, she said:

"I'm aware of the general situation here, Katie. This must be extremely difficult for you. Before you go on, please know that you don't need to tell me anything."

"Thank you," I said, "but I'd like to." With the words spoken aloud, I suddenly realised the depth of their truth: I wanted – needed – someone trustworthy to know every last detail, as in reality, it was so much harder to continue to keep it all inside.

"I had been in bed when Dad shouted at me to come downstairs. I could tell by his panicked tone that something was very wrong. It was me who called the ambulance; Dad had been too busy trying to sort her out. And then, suddenly, I was in the house alone. Adrenalin quickly took over and I was on auto-pilot. Dad had gone ahead in the ambulance with Mum. Nausea swept over me, along with a frantic sense of the need to organise – to make everything alright again, to bring order back to chaos. I dragged Mum's bag downstairs, which I'd packed full of her things. For a moment, I tried to convince myself that she was just going away on holiday. But, tricking myself was impossible – she would have no control over how long she'd be gone. It may be weeks or even months. My heart pounded in my chest and my ears rang with the sound of blood pumping at high-speed. It felt as if there was an angel and a demon arguing in my head over whether to take the car or not. It was only a week until I'd be legal to drive. *Who would know?* But I thought I might get caught or have an accident and that would only make things much worse for Mum. So instead, I managed to run what felt like miles to the hospital, carrying her stuffed overnight bag."

I paused to take a sip of tea and, as I placed the cup to my lips, I realized that the incessant shaking had all but stopped. A feeling of inner calmness welled inside of me as I continued to articulate, for the first time, the previous week's surreal events. My headmistress sat before me in patient silence, as if she had all the time in the world. I pretty much knew her reality was the complete opposite; but also, that she seemed to understand how badly I'd needed this outlet. Talking about it felt like a "now or never" situation – and something inside me knew that now was by far the healthiest option of the two.

Over the next hour, I described everything that happened after I'd staggered breathlessly into the emergency room. The way my head felt light, almost disconnected, as if I was watching someone else's life unfold. *Maybe I had died and was viewing the scene from above?* – at least, it felt safer to think that way. Still panting from my long run with the bag, I'd slowly walked over to the figure lying on the bed in the centre of the treatment room. She looked like my mum; but, at the same time, seemed strangely unfamiliar. *How could a person I thought was indestructible look so helpless and pathetic?* I felt betrayed, angry and then guilty for feeling such a mish-mash of disallowed emotions. My eyes locked onto the soaked bandages covering her wrists and the scratches on her neck. But it was the sight of the blood-soaked patch on her chest, just above her heart, that made my head swim. Before I could faint, I raced to the door to fill my lungs with fresh air. Instantly, I felt reconnected with everyday reality as I hugged my knees for comfort, focusing on simple, concrete things, around which I could easily wrap my brain; the feel of the cold stone step numbing my backside, the warmth of the summer day just coming alive, ants crawling across the pavement, birds calling to each other across the wires above my head.

Shortly after I'd braved it back inside, Mum was moved to the psychiatric ward; but not before one of the attending nurses politely took me aside.

"Would you like this back?" she said, holding out the knife my mum had used to stab herself. I stared at it in her hand. Cleared of Mum's blood and wrapped in a plastic bag, it looked like any ordinary kitchen knife; however, the thought of ever chopping my vegetables with it again wasn't something I could comprehend.

"No, thank you," I managed to politely reply, as I faked a weak smile. Inside, I felt an overwhelming urge to scream a litany of obscenities at this insensitive creature. *Why, the fuck, would I ever want this thing back?* As she shrugged and walked away, I instantly berated myself. *Good God, I'm a terrible person. She's only doing her job and it's probably protocol to return all property. Why couldn't I just have taken the knife and made her feel better about herself?*

I spent the rest of the day being quizzed by doctors, all keen for Mum to speak, although she wasn't saying a word. Not even to Dad or me.

"How long has she been feeling suicidal?"

"No idea," we both responded, looking at each other blankly. Again, my internal reaction was worlds away from what I'd said aloud. *How the hell should I know?* I wanted to shout at them. *What mother actually talks about such things with her child?* And, it would be true – ever since her attempt with the slug pellets when I was just a baby, the whole issue of Mum's fragile mental state had effectively been glossed over; anesthetised by Mum's laundry list of anti-psychotic medication, as well as by her exhaustive efforts to rise above their debilitating side-effects, and what remained of her very secret, inner turmoil, which the medication couldn't seem to touch. Even at just seventeen, it seemed painfully obvious to me that when someone is doing everything they can to create a "normal" world for themselves and their family, the last thing they're going to do is admit to dwelling in a cavernous, seemingly irreparable pit of suicidal despair in a society that interprets such feelings as insanity.

When I'd finally finished telling my headmistress every detail of my family's darkest secret, we sat in silence for a moment.

"I'm so sorry, Katie," she finally muttered. It was really

such a generic thing to say; yet, I felt incredible gratitude towards her. For, in her simple willingness to listen, she had provided greater validation than I had ever received from anyone in my life. I hadn't had to pretend I was "fine" when I was anything but.

Outside, the sun was beginning to set and long, cool shadows fell across the tiled kitchen. As I got up to leave, I didn't know what the future would bring. I didn't know if I'd pass or fail my French exam; or any exams actually. I didn't know if my life would ever be "normal". Thankfully, I also didn't know that my mum would remain sectioned for many months to come. Everything felt completely beyond my control. I could only hope and pray that Mum would be back to us soon, whole and finally healed by the doctors into whose hands my father and I had been forced to entrust her. It was a helpless feeling; yet, as my headmistress sent me off with a warm, consolatory hug – one that would have left most of my fellow pupils speechless – a small inkling of wisdom began to dawn that, even in a world spiralling so out-of-control, I could at least feel empowered by speaking my truth. For the first time in a week, I felt a glimmer of hope as I left her house, my "summoning" having served a vastly different purpose than "judgement". *I shouldn't have judged her.* At the time, it was only a pinprick of understanding, but enough to know that holding-in secrets and maintaining brave fronts was a toxic endeavour, which only served to generate even more (unnecessary) pain and guilt than I already carried.

To this day, I still look back with great appreciation for the kindness and compassion my headmistress showed me when I'd needed it most. And, if there was any real-life version of a "mystical creature waiting at the top of the stairs" – as in that old, childhood dream – perhaps, it was the simple yet profound presence of Truth. The Truth can be scary to approach, but once the door is open, the welcome is comforting. The starkness of this realisation dared me to hope – just a little – that one day, there would be a way out of the "madness" that had always plagued my family. For now, such normality was only a dream – but at least the door had been cracked open. Who knew what magical, mystical experiences the future may bring.

FOUR

A SECURE SIGH OF RELIEF

Your environment influences who you become;
be mindful of your surroundings.

Looking back, I suppose that Erving Goffman's book
*Asylums: Essays on the Social Situation of Mental Patients
& Other Inmates* was a rather unusual request from a
teenager on the brink of leaving high school. While most of
my friends cared more about which pubs they were going to
party at after the presentation ceremony, I couldn't wait to
devour the modest literary award our school customarily
offered as a reward for achieving A-Level grades. I prayed
that the unusually insightful book would contain the
answers to my most important questions. Top of the list, I
wanted to know what the hell had happened to my mum,
and why the bloody doctors still refused to let her come
home. It had been months and she still only spent the
occasional weekend with us, pacing around the kitchen,
seemingly distraught but unable to express why. Not that her
lengthy hospital stay hadn't been understandable, at least
to some degree; after all, she had tried to stab herself in the
heart, whilst making strange allegations that she hadn't
actually done it herself. I don't know how close to fatal her
injuries had been on that horrible morning, but her grisly

wounds had certainly been life-destroying, if not life-threatening. Yet, no matter how many months of hospitalization, emotion-numbing medication, and brutal electro-convulsive treatment she endured, Mum never wavered from her well-vocalized belief that she'd been momentarily possessed at the time by some unknown, evil spirit; for her, the decision to pick up that knife and do the unthinkable had been completely beyond her control. Dad and I could never bring ourselves to discuss whether or not such a supernatural atrocity was possible; I think we both just assumed her blaming an evil entity was just another sign that she was seriously ill. And truthfully, we didn't want to think any other reason could be to blame: the only thing worse than knowing one's own mother was capable of inflicting such wounds upon herself, was the idea of an evil spirit having that kind of horrific power. At the time, I simply couldn't even go there.

Somewhat reluctantly, I joined everyone in their non-stop pub celebrations, smiling happily for the many, commemorative photos that were taken to mark what should have been a very auspicious occasion; while inside, barely feeling anything beyond the webbing of distrust and despair that had effectively entangled my soul.

A few, fleeting months later, I stood with my parents in front of the University of Bradford in Yorkshire, ready to meet the promising new social and academic worlds that lay before me. Mum had only recently been released from hospital; and both outwardly and inwardly, she was decidedly a different person. Not only was she dealing with the severe effects of her anti-psychotic cocktail, which made it difficult for her to relax or feel much emotion, the lengthy hospital stay had also proved to be quite emaciating. My once healthily voluptuous mum now swam in her oversized clothing, although, surprisingly, she didn't seem to notice.

She did her best to try to hide it, but the stress and sadness of having to send her only child off to university showed easily in the pain behind her eyes. Given the circumstances, such feelings were only natural for any mother; but mine also had to bear the brunt of knowing she was under constant scrutiny for each and every emotional reaction she had. What was not promptly medicated away must have been hard for her to handle. I'm sure she often found herself self-consciously wondering if she should let what was left of her emotions show, or keep the contents of her heart concealed from the harsh judgement of others. And so she remained frozen in a fear that affected not only her, but everyone close to her. This lack of outward affection, plus the horrendous guilt I felt at leaving my Dad to deal with the worry alone, played heavy on my crumbling heart.

Neither of my parents had any last-minute advice as they helped me get settled into my tiny, one-person dorm room; no doubt they were frozen in the knowledge that I wouldn't listen anyway; I was emotionally frozen and snappy myself. They dutifully followed me into the large, community kitchen three floors down to put away my dishes and a few left-overs they'd brought from home. Mum and Dad were simple, small town folk, unaccustomed to the sights and sounds of a big University campus. With the exception of my Dad making silly attempts at jokes and being overly-chatty with other students, the hustle and bustle of this kitchen metropolis, with all of its diversity and city-speak, seemed to completely overwhelm Mum's senses.

"You planning on starting a plastic container business?" joked a young man from behind the newspaper he was reading, sitting at the kitchen table.

"Thinking about it," I replied, returning his wry smile with a roll of my eyes towards my parents. At that very moment, the bulging carrier bag holding the empty containers split open, and old margarine tubs clattered all over the floor.

I could feel my cheeks instantly flush to scarlet as the four of us dove to opposite ends of the stained tile floor to pick them up. "Why on earth did you pack all of these?" I asked my parents, somewhat severely.

"We thought you could store your leftovers in them, love," my Dad retorted, beaming his ever-present smile at me.

"Okay. You can go now if you like. I'll manage. Thanks," I said, trying to maintain a sliver of cool nonchalance in front of this friendly, inarguably attractive stranger who didn't seem to mind helping out. There was gentleness in his dark brown eyes that somehow made him look calm and sure of himself, even safe, all of which I found really appealing.

For a moment, Mum and Dad looked awkwardly at me and at each other. Then, Dad gave me a bear hug that was tight enough to nearly collapse my lungs. Mum's hug, on the

41

other hand, felt like a limp, half-hearted, token gesture. I knew that her drugs were what made her act so robotically; still, I desperately wanted her to show me that she loved me. In the back of my mind, I couldn't help wondering if she blamed me, at least a little, for everything awful that had happened since my birth. I certainly blamed myself and I needed to be forgiven.

As I watched them drive away, part of me was laden with guilt over the fact that I would not be there anymore to keep my mum safe, while another, previously unknown, part of me relished in a sudden surge of relief and freedom. I had consistently been the "strong" one during the eighteen months that my mother had been hospitalized. I hadn't realized how exhausting that role truly was, until I finally found myself alone in my shoebox of a dorm room, with only my books, clothes, and the sound of my own breathing to keep me company. Immediately, I found such silence somewhat uncomfortable and quickly second-guessed how much I'd really enjoy being on my own. I didn't want time to stop and think, my thoughts weren't nice and I needed a distraction from them.

For better or for worse, my new-found solitude did not last very long. That night, a group of us, including the helpful, young man from the kitchen debacle, all went out for a curry together. We spent the first week at University drinking and partying as it was "Fresher's week". I found myself instantly drawn to "Mr Plastic Container". I could tell him anything – even the details of the nightmare with my mum – and he quickly became my rock, offering consistency and security in a tumultuous, unknown world. I hadn't been looking for a boyfriend, but our friendship quickly blossomed. Everyone believed us to be the perfect couple; and, on the surface, they were right. We never argued about anything and he fitted seamlessly into my family. My parents – relieved I'd met someone and found the "security" they'd wanted for my future – treated him like the son they'd never had. I'd always longed for emotional trust and stability; and now, here it was, as if presented on a silver platter. And really, what could offer more promise, more hope, more reasons to rebuild the foundations of my crumbling heart than the abiding love and loyalty of a kind and decent man?

FIVE

FOR BETTER OR WORSE

*Your body speaks your mind; it could be fatal not
to listen to what it may be trying to tell you.*

I'd been planning my "fairy-tale" wedding for almost
eighteen months, distracting myself from a general sense of
unfathomable unease by diving headfirst into a sea of pre-
wedding details, most of which felt rather frivolous and
unnecessarily expensive. With each dress–fitting, and when
I pondered over flower and music choice, I became more
desperate to experience the kind of soul-fulfilling happiness
modern society makes brides-to-be believe they should feel.
It shouldn't have been so hard; after all, I had a lovely, doting
fiancé and was heading towards the secure future I'd always
wanted. Marriage represented everything I had imagined
for myself; therefore, my puzzling lack of genuine
enthusiasm added immense guilt to an already topsy-turvy
emotional equation. At least trying-on bridal gowns seemed
to keep my mum happy. And, that's what I wanted to do
most of all – please everybody else around me. Everything
would be okay, as long as the people I loved kept smiling.

Mysteriously, as my wedding day drew nearer and my
desperation to lose as much weight as possible grew
stronger, running became progressively more difficult, as if

I was twenty stone and dragging myself through porridge. Why was I so lethargic all the time?

Work had also grown increasingly laborious, as I drove every day to a deprived area in the South Wales valleys to help people who were depressed and unable to help themselves. *At least, I wasn't anything like them.* Many of my clients were on the verge of homelessness, penniless, lonely, and dealing with a multitude of illnesses, most of which were obviously emotionally initiated. As for my own "unhealthy" state; the cause continued to elude me. Certainly, my problems were vastly different than my clients. Any sickness I experienced was probably simply due to a virus I'd picked up somewhere along the way. I just needed to "ride it out" and, perhaps, double up on my intake of vitamin C and iron.

Over the coming months, I managed this way – in what could best be described as a "head-in-the-sand" state. However, when I could no longer find a speck of humour in the most common, inarguably humorous scenarios – when merely chuckling at clever office banter seemed to drain my already-depleted energy supplies – I finally knew it was time to seek the help of a professional. Although I usually loved being behind the wheel, the drive from work to the surgery seemed like a slog. I could barely hold my head up behind the wheel. The clinic was perched up on a hill, and as I surveyed the scene below, I suddenly felt an overwhelming urge to pull over onto the verge.

Resting my clammy forehead on the soft rubber steering wheel, I vividly remember the heat from a reservoir of stored tears as they finally escaped down my cheeks, dripping salty confusion onto my trembling knees. What the hell was wrong with me? I wiped my eyes, blew my nose, and dug deep for a revival of energy to simply get myself to the doctor's office. Once in the waiting room, I dithered between thoughts about why I hadn't taken this step sooner, and what the hell I was doing here. Previously, when I'd felt this listless, the darkness had blessedly passed after making a modestly concerted effort to take things a bit more slowly. *Maybe I was just pitiful.* After all, how could someone who led such a healthy lifestyle' someone so blessed with love and a world of creature comforts, really, truly be suffering? Lots of people suffered far worse things. Endless masses the world over endured far more agonizing circumstances and conditions than some vague sense of general malaise felt by a whining twenty-something on the verge of "happily ever after".

What possible right did I have to even complain?

"Miss Mottram, the doctor will see you now," the receptionist called. *Well, it was clearly too late to turn back now.*

Timidly, I entered the general practitioner's office, and immediately took stock of the shadowy, cluttered room. It reminded me of an archaic bachelor pad, brimming with dark, stuffy-looking leather furniture, and stagnant air that smelled of sweat and hair grease. "Take a seat, love. What can I do for you?"

As I obediently rattled off my list of symptoms, my mouth felt so dry, I virtually needed to spit out the words. I could feel my cheeks instantly flush as I shrank smaller and smaller into the leather wing chair. Reminding myself that this was an important man whose help I'd enlisted, I worked hard to mask the discomfort I felt from simply being in his presence. Any uneasiness I felt was obviously my problem. Self-blame came easy to me, as usual.

"So you're getting married in a few weeks, you say?"

"Yes, I ..."

"Huh," his leering eyes bore into me, raising an eyebrow as he interrupted. "It seems to me like you need to go and sleep around a bit. Make sure that you're doing the right thing."

Did I actually hear that right? Immediately, I sensed something very predatorial in the air. A bead of sweat ran down my forehead. I felt like shouting at this "doctor", sitting there all high and mighty on his fancy, swivel throne. *Who the fuck did he think he was, saying something so wildly inappropriate to a complete stranger?* To a female patient, no less. But instead, I kept quiet. He was the expert, as was formidably emphasised by the elaborately-framed plaques decorating the walls behind him, each clearly having added an extra bit of plumage to his already overly puffed-up chest. Sufficiently intimidated, I smiled sweetly and pretended to laugh off his offensive comment.

"I think we'd better do a blood test, just to make sure there's nothing more than a virus going on here," he announced, leading me into the back room and commanding that I lay down on the treatment bed. I didn't divulge that I hated needles with a passion. Now, the only thing on equal par to my distain for needles was how much I disliked this sharp, foul little man with a giant-sized ego. The pinprick itself didn't really hurt, but the pent-up anxiety and subsequent relief at it being over suddenly overpowered me enough that I blacked out. When I came around a few minutes later, I was relieved to see a kindly-looking female nurse bent over me, fanning my face.

"Can I give you a lift home?" the doctor casually offered, staring at me long enough to further unnerve me, even in the presence of the attending nurse. "You probably shouldn't be driving in your condition."

My condition? Too afraid to even probe into what he felt that might be – other than a lack of sexual conquests – I managed to curtly say, "I'm fine. I'll just call my husband-to-be."

After a short wait for the blood to completely return to my head, my fiancé appeared at the office and escorted me back to the safety of our little home. As I stepped through the door, I was immediately greeted by a wagging tail and unconditional kisses from my other love, Vinnie, the rescue Beagle. Back in familiar surroundings, my relief felt truly palpable, and I suddenly realised that I must indeed be making solid choices. What a scary thought to be "out there" on the search for security in such clearly shark-infested waters. Feeling safe and loved by a devoted, gentle man was comforting, illness or no illness. Furthermore, I'd been raised to believe that happiness – for women at least – was contingent on marriage, security and children. The elated feeling I'd read all brides should experience may thus far have eluded me; but at least, I finally knew that I was on the right path, surrounded by all the necessary ingredients to find happiness. It was only a matter of time until the recipe brought forth said happiness as a constant, sustainable emotion that mirrored the many, wonderful blessings I so obviously took for granted.

SIX

DÉJÀ-VU

"Have I gone mad?" asked the Mad Hatter. "I'm
afraid so," said Alice, "You're entirely bonkers.
But I'll tell you a secret. All the best people are."

LEWIS CARROLL

I watched her from the window end of the family room although she was oblivious to my gaze. The warmth I was feeling was radiating from the heater on which I was perched, there was none radiating from her. The only noise was that of the news bulletins on half volume in the background, and the incessant tapping of her foot on the lino floor. Her hair was greasy and dishevelled, and she was wearing that bloody old jumper again – the one with the owls on the front she said was lucky – as if it was a compulsory, stale uniform. Suddenly she turned towards me and my heart skipped a beat, I felt the urge to spread myself across the window commando-style, just in case she thought she could fly and tried to jump out. But my feet stayed firmly wedged, I mustn't show any sign of panic.

"I knew you'd come", she said, dead seriously. "I've been watching you on the telly and I've been expecting you in the helicopter." I stifled an uncomfortable smirk, and wished I had a tape recorder, she'd never believe what she said when I recounted her words to her later.

As she heavily slept off the effects of the Risperidone I guiltily slipped away again, leaving her in the care of the night staff, hardened over the years from so much repressed emotion of their own, petrified of letting anyone see a chink in their perfectly sane armour. I knew that uniform well; I wore it to work myself now, there was no other way to survive.

I was shattered after the six-hour rally drive over from Wales just a few hours earlier, in a frantic state following a frustrating telephone exchange with Dad:

"She's acting really strangely again, panting as if she's giving birth."

"Have you phoned the doctor? It sounds like she needs to go back into hospital." I'd retorted, all self-righteous with my insider knowledge.

"Oh she'll be alright in the morning." *Yeah, right. Pull your head out of the sand, Dad.* Except I hadn't actually dared to say that of course. So to whom was my anger directed? Mum for having another "episode" at such an inconvenient time when I should have been at work, or Dad, for not having dealt with the situation in the way in which I wanted? Or maybe it was at myself, for being so resentful about something that was really nobody's fault. None of this would be happening if I hadn't been born.

It was ten o'clock when I finally flopped into bed. And I was laying there, in the room, in which I used to play, once so happily unaware of the complexities of adult life, wishing that I was back there, in that "unreality" of my childhood.

My brain, clearly needing to process my desire to regress, was actively dreaming.

She shouted to me from downstairs;

"Tea's almost ready".

"Okay, I'll be down in a minute," I yell, already packing away Sindy, separate to Paul, just to make sure they can't reproduce in the night. Now that I know how it could happen it must be prevented, I don't want mini plastic babies taking over the order of the playroom. I bounce downstairs two at a time, and then climb back up and jump to the floor, first from one step, then from two, until I get to eight and can't manage anymore without risking a lifetime of paralysis. Why? Who cares? That's the sort of mindless stupid thing kids do and nobody bats an eyelid. At what point does it become socially unacceptable to have mindless fun? As I sprint into the kitchen and skid along the lino in my socks, I spot Nan sitting at the table. She's grinding her teeth as usual, but it's not that that startles me, (she'd not be the same with two full front teeth), it's her mere presence. I'd forgotten she was coming for tea today. Who needs routine when you're ten years old? I go over and give her a squeeze, and she smiles her goofy disconnected smile as she hugs me back and I sit down beside her.

"What time will Dad be home?" I ask to the room in general.

"No telling, he's got a late job on," Mum sighs. She knows, as I do, that he'll be stressed and uptight when he gets in. Her cheeks are glowing from the steam the potatoes are giving off as she mashes them with gusto. The smell of melted butter wafts under my nose and my mouth begins to water as she brings the plates over – the dutiful housewife in her plastic pinny adorned with Minnie Mouse. There are still traces of burnt condensed cream on Minnie's face from the time the pan boiled dry and Mum didn't quite get to it in time before it exploded all over the kitchen. We sit in silence, eating in contemplation, three generations of quietly sensitive philosophisers. About what we were philosophising, none of us were really sure, but from an outsiders perspective, we would have had the same glint in our eyes.

The loud "whoosh" of the back door opening as Dad returned home in my dream, woke me from my actual half-sleep. I stretched out and rolled over, desperately trying to get back to sleep and escape again into happier times. But it was no good, my bladder and brain refused to let me rest. I reluctantly dragged myself from under the safety of the duvet and felt my way in the dark, along to the bathroom. As I pulled the cord the sudden bright light caused me to squint in the same way as if I were in the spotlight in the middle of a dark stage, and I felt strangely exposed in the same way. The mirror appeared to have been invaded by someone who insisted at staring back at me, frighteningly aged over the last few years, with huge bags under their eyes in desperate need of unpacking. I decided to skip the fight with sleep and went downstairs to make a cup of tea instead, tea was supposed to cure anything. *Why, at twenty-six, was I so scared of being alone in the kitchen at night? Was I afraid that the demons that took over Mum that summer's morning nine years previously would take over me too?* It was always in these moments that I seemed to remember the unexplained eeriness of the knowledge of the clairvoyant I had once visited with Mum. He had known about things that he had no other way of knowing. *If spirits were only a figment of our imagination how did he say they had told him things that were actually true?* It was too spooky. As I opened the cutlery drawer to get out a teaspoon, my eyes were drawn to the space which would have still held the chopping knife of doom, (if that really tactful nurse had had her way), and shivers coursed their way down my spine.

The next morning I woke, still tired from a restless night of ups and downs and dreams about running with legs of lead and ghosts that were trying to talk to me. After a breakfast of pretend normality with Dad, we returned to the ward where the staff now knew us on first name terms. Dad bantered with them as we walked down the corridor, we were quite the little double-act, not really realising at the time how reliant we were on each other's faked ability to cope.

"Morning, Mum," I said cheerily as I sat down by her side in the dining room, "how are you feeling today?" The panic in her eyes really struck me that morning; I hadn't really noticed previously how petrified she was of being in the hospital; maybe I hadn't wanted to see.

"Better," she replied, "but they keep lying about what I was doing yesterday, saying I was doing things I know I'd never do, making out I'm mad."

I felt like laughing, but not because it was funny. Even I didn't know what was real and what wasn't anymore. *Was I going mad too?* After all it was supposed to be hereditary. *So what if I was?* There was nothing I could do about it, and anyway, I spent enough time at work preaching about what a thin line there is between sanity and insanity;

"It's all socially dictated" I'd state, trying to reduce the stigma. But did I really know what I meant when I said that? And if it was all organically "normal" and acceptable to me, why was I so scared that I could be about to cross the line? Or maybe I had and nobody had noticed yet. All that could be done, was to carry on and hide the fact that I was struggling to cope, for everybody else's sake. Thank goodness for the safety of my little chocolate-box life, to which I could retreat.

That evening I drove back to Wales. Distancing myself physically from the chaos made it somehow easier to cope, emotionally. *Maybe if I carried on driving it would all go away?*

SEVEN

SECOND CHANCES AND SELF-AWARENESS

*"You've always had the power my dear,
you just had to learn it for yourself."*
GLINDA, WIZARD OF OZ. L. FRANK BAUM.

"Did you get a chance to finish your homework today?" I asked the young girl slumped miserably in the passenger seat next to me, as I drove her back to the children's therapeutic community at which I'd been working for the past nine months.

My husband had accepted a job in Norfolk, which meant moving back closer to my parents; at least it served to reduce the guilt I felt deep down at being so far away. I wanted to keep my distance because it made the pain easier to bear, but I was confused and ashamed whenever I remotely thought about prioritising my own desires. The voice of another well-meaning nurse rang in my ears whenever I dreamt about staying away; "Your mum would love it if you moved back closer to home, she really needs you, you know", she had said to me during my last visit to the ward. I'd easily managed to get myself another job; having moved around the mental health field so much meant that I had gained wide experience, which really seemed to pay off in interviews. My succession of different jobs over the last few years had clearly resulted from my attempts to cure a perpetual itch of dissatisfaction.

"Fuck off," the girl snapped back in response, keeping her eyes on the road ahead. "Sort out your own life before you try to sort out everyone else's!"

Gripping the steering wheel so tight that I could feel my shoulders tense, I reminded myself that my twelve-year-old passenger was a needy, emotionally distraught child – one who's own mother couldn't care for her due to her own emotional distress, no less – who had endured a lifetime of turmoil in her barely dozen years. Still, it took all my inner strength to remain calm and not immediately snap back. In general, this field of work had proved to be an extremely challenging experience. From the minute I'd taken the job as children's key worker, I'd not only felt my patience continually being tested, but also found it necessary to hide the volatile see-saw of emotions I inexplicably experienced from both my new colleagues and the young clients, for whose support I'd been assigned. It was an exhausting ordeal; but apparently, I hadn't been as good at masking my pent-up feelings as I'd thought. Resisting a sudden, irrational impulse to run the car off the road, something which I was considering with increasing frequency when alone recently, I ignored the girl's rudeness and focused on getting her safely back to the house, where I could immediately pass her off to co-workers who didn't have time to psycho-analyse my inner turmoil. For that, I was immensely grateful, as I seemed to be riding a rollercoaster of unsettled, haunted feelings that validated this young girl's caustic, off-handed remark much more than I was ready to admit.

Although I hadn't been able to pinpoint the exact source of my disquiet, it had begun to manifest itself in recurring and very painful bouts of kidney infections. On one hand, the infections were a complete pain in the arse (or, more specifically, in the lower back); but, on the other hand, the time off work they required me to take felt like a welcomed reprieve. At least when I was at home recuperating, I didn't have to battle to suppress the sheer, debilitating anxiety that arose each time I approached the long drive at the beginning of a shift. Why was I so afraid, and of what exactly? I was the adult, after all; the one in control who was there to offer support to the poor, little mites who had ended up alone and at the mercy of total strangers, clearly petrified and in desperate need of love and security. My job – interacting with the children, and rewarding and disciplining their behaviour – seemed simple enough; yet I struggled endlessly to stay "above" the true depth of their pain. There was something about their collective despair that felt hardwired directly into my own, as if it were a metal pick tapping on a rotting tooth. It was all I could do to keep the "infection" of repressed sorrow contained to a small, manageable section of my brain; but, now, with my kidneys reacting severely as well, I knew that it was only a matter of time before I was fully "contaminated". And, while a tooth could eventually be extracted, I had no idea how I'd ever begin to successfully remove the kind of deep-rooted agony that seemed to be slowly seeping its way through both my body and mind.

A few days later, Miss "Fuck Off" was in the middle of one of her daily tantrums, screaming obscenities at my colleagues who were trying to hold her down in a textbook restraint, as she punched and spit angrily at them. Whilst they calmly asked her to stop, repeatedly telling her that she was safe, I could feel her transferred terror course its way through my own veins, making my heart race and my eyes moist with tears. Immediately, she shot me a look across the room that seemed to sear straight through me.

"You're pathetic," she snarled, seizing onto my emotional vulnerability like a predator that enjoyed playing with its cornered prey. "Get a grip of yourself!"

Even though the medically-trained, rational side of me knew exactly why this girl had targeted me – my teary-eyed vulnerability meant that I didn't pose a threat – I couldn't help but take her piercing words to heart. My stomach fluttered from the combination of genuine love and pity I felt towards this poor child who had suffered so deeply, along with a strong wave of shame, helplessness, and self-loathing. She may have been only twelve, but this time, I couldn't deny the hard, cold truth behind her angry words. *Why wasn't I stronger? How was it possible to feel such a tidal wave of conflicting emotions simultaneously washing over me and remain afloat?*

Later that day, when things had quieted back into a

relatively "normal" routine, the staff sat with the children around the dinner table enjoying a delicious tea-time spread. It was customary during such afternoon teas for the children to choose a staff member to spend fifteen minutes of pre-bedtime settling with them that coming evening. To my surprise, for the first time ever Miss "Fuck Off" chose me. A wave of nausea swept over me as I imagined her continuing her personal attack in the privacy of her own room. However, despite my inner desire to recoil, I put on my very best poker face, smiling as I politely thanked her for her decision to choose me.

Just before lights out, I knocked gently on the girl's door and asked if it was okay to come in. When I entered, I found her sprawled on the carpet in her baggy T-shirt and football shorts, busily preoccupied with an impressive collection of drawings she'd created. A multitude of brightly coloured, felt-tipped pens lay strewn on the floor all around her, creating a cautionary, makeshift barrier from the outside world.

"Hi," she mumbled to me quietly, glancing up quickly before resuming her thoughtfully-placed strokes on the page. Her drawings were meticulous and precise and full of richly colourful details. I could scarcely believe this was the girl who had been screaming and lashing out earlier that day. Slowly, I sat down on the scratchy carpet in front of her, being extra careful to stay just outside of her rainbow-pen barricade.

"What are you drawing?" I asked.

"It's my invention," she said, somewhat shyly. "See these?" She pointed to one of the pictures. "They're turbo-charged football boots that give you special, speedy powers on the pitch."

I smiled, and suddenly felt my whole being – body and mind – begin to deeply relax for the first time in weeks. Deep down, beneath the tough, spiteful exterior, there was something about this young girl that sparkled with incredible potential. Just as I was thinking of it, an image of one of my closest friends from high school flashed vividly through my mind's eye. My friend, also named Katie, had died from a malignant brain tumour shortly after we'd graduated from university. Although Katie's passing had happened years ago, I still occasionally felt her presence nearly as strongly as I did when she was alive. Perhaps it was just the dear, bittersweet memory of her and her uncanny ability to always remain so positive and full of warmth, sparkle, and charisma, right up to the very end. Regardless, I couldn't help but think of Katie now, drawing on her beautiful energy that seemed to defy death and wondering what she would say to this girl, if given the opportunity. *She needs to know that life is trying hard to give her a second chance, Katie; that she can still have a long and happy road ahead of her, regardless of the pain of the past. All it takes is the ability to trust again. To forgive and to believe, most of all in herself. She needs to know that it's safe to trust, in order to let down her defences that keep her so isolated.*

"That's so cool," I finally said aloud, sucking in a long,

deep breath. Was it actually possible that Katie's spirit was with me? I remembered how, during her funeral, I'd watched as a solitary, brilliantly-hued butterfly had slowly made its way through the entire sanctuary of the crowded church, alighting softly on the shoulders of dozens of mourners before turning to flutter back outdoors. Later, as Katie's grief-stricken mother had entered her house, she'd distinctly heard the notes of a familiar song that had been played earlier that day as Katie's coffin was carried through the congregation, emanating from the stereo in the lounge;

"Angels" by Robbie Williams filled her ears.

But the stereo hadn't been switched on.

Despite my lack of spirituality at the time, and hesitancy to believe in anything that wasn't completely "logical", I couldn't help but internally play with the idea that, yes, such things were entirely possible. After all, I had been privy to my own mum's slightly abnormal, (and scary), beliefs that spirits could absolutely continue to communicate with us after their physical bodies had ceased to be. *If everything was energy, and energy couldn't disappear, then wasn't it logical that nothing ever actually ceased to exist?* It was all so confusing, I'd rather just not think about it.

Turning my full attention back to the young subject that had initiated these deep musings, I quickly added,

"Those boots would be awesome to have. But really, I don't think you need any special powers. I've seen you play and you look pretty amazing without any extra help. But hey, maybe they'd be useful for the other players?"

She looked up and, for the very first time, beamed widely and hopefully at me; her deep, sea-green eyes easily speaking a thousand words. For the next, few minutes, we talked about her favourite sports, and I told her that I'd just started yoga classes and found them quite good fun. She asked me what yoga was, and so I demonstrated a silly-looking position, getting her to join in until she fell about laughing. In that moment, I knew that she had sensed I'd needed to make a connection that day too. Allowing me in to her private world of drawings, hopes, and dreams had been her way of apologising to me for her angry words. Even in her desperately needy state, she had been aware of my sadness, which seemed amazing to me. We exchanged another smile, and in those precious few seconds, I felt a deep connection with this girl, as if we truly understood each other on a soulful level.

As I bid the young girl good-night, I wondered how many soulful moments like this it would take before she could finally feel safe enough to release that protective, venomous side once and for all. Clearly, this child had the potential to make a truly positive impact on her world, if only she would be willing to give herself the second chance she deserved. In my mind, I could easily recall the distinctly contagious giggle of my friend, Katie, a girl with a penchant for all things pink, and a sunny, irrepressible zest for life that made it incomprehensible as to why hers had been cut so horrifically short. Yet, somehow, Katie's essence was still here, providing the gentle, fluttering guidance I'd needed to realise that –

even during times of overwhelming and intractable pain – human connection on a soulful level didn't need to be logical; the benefits it offered outweighed anything the brain could possibly comprehend.

EIGHT

POTENTIAL NEW BEGINNINGS

Never attach your happiness to anything,
because a "thing" can be taken away

Between my shifts and a busy married life, interspersed with endorphin-inducing runs, I thankfully had little time to focus on any gnawing sense of unease. And then, two years later, this time happily settled into yet another job, I was blessed with what I considered to be a vital ingredient for happiness in the symbol of two, clear, pink lines on a plastic stick. My heart sang and fluttered with a combination of excitement and nervousness. That night, I allowed myself to dream about the prospect of becoming a good mother myself, reflecting on the connection I had been able to make with the children at the home a couple of years previously, despite my own inner turmoil. I felt as if the life I'd envisioned was finally working out exactly the way I'd always hoped.

A few days later, I awoke to a bitterly-cold morning; overnight, everything for miles around had been blanketed in a sparkling layer of frost. My breath hung like enchanted mist as I made my way out to my car, carefully taking extra small steps on the slippery pavement. The "warm glow" inside didn't help to heat my extremities, so I blasted my little Smart car's heater before setting off for the office, blowing into my hands in order to get the blood recirculating. In my head, I imagined the moment I would tell my colleagues that I was going to have a baby. There would be hugs and smiles, and unspoken concern that in a few months' time they'd be down a member of staff. They would certainly cope just fine. I knew this from experience, as the previous year I had needed to take a few weeks off for yet another bout of ambiguous illness. When I'd expressed my guilt over my absence, my manager had told me, matter-of-factly:

"This place will hardly fall apart if you're not here, Katie."

The words had stung, but they were true enough. At least, taking time off for having a baby wasn't a reason I'd feel guilty about. I was ever-conscious that within me grew a uniquely precious gift for not only my husband and I, but also for my parents. This one, tiny child-in-the-making would not make its appearance for months, but she (or he) had already opened up a whole, new "baby-oriented" promise of happiness the four of us could happily discuss, plan for, and anticipate with collective excitement.

Just a few, short miles from the office, the gently winding road glistened brightly in the reflection of my headlights. As a precaution, I gently tapped my brakes; but, instead of slowing, the tiny car skidded sideways and then backwards, while my still-cold hands made desperate attempts to steady the wheel and my feet danced with ineffectual pedals. In a flash, the idea of regaining control became futile. After what felt like a triple spin, my Smart car slammed sideways into the unforgiving trunk of a large oak tree, its plastic bodywork folding as sharply as a bent spoon around it, as my own body slammed hard against the steering column. For a few minutes, I sat there, feeling shell-shocked. Then, with legs like jelly, I shakily opened the door and tried to get my bearings. It was only then that I noticed how ominous the tree-lined road – now more of a skating rink of thick black ice – had become. After unsteadily dialling my husband's phone number my hands immediately went to cover my womb as my mind flooded with a tidal wave of dread.

I spent the next five days following strict doctor's orders to stay in bed, as I waited for an ultrasound appointment which would determine if my baby had survived the crash. Naturally, the waiting wreaked havoc on my mental state. I spent the entire time alternately crying over the possibility that my dream of motherhood had been shattered along with my car, and trying not to move, having developed a rather irrational fear that even a very deep breath may potentially cause the baby further damage. At least, my breath was something I could control. By the end of what felt like the longest five days of my life, my emotional state had plummeted beyond exhaustion, and I had developed an intimate knowledge of every lump and bump of paint on the bedroom ceiling.

Finally, the day of the scan had arrived and I found myself lying on the table in the maternity ward of my local hospital. Resignedly, I held out my arm for another needle prick that, along with the scan, would reveal my baby's viability. Funny how relative fear is—where I had once considered needles to be the scariest thing in the world, I now felt them nothing compared to the prospect of a crumbled dream and the loss of a tiny life I may never know. A small part of me clung to a sliver of hope, even though my gut told me with no uncertainty, that it was time to let my baby go. The bleeding following the crash had been substantial. Looking at those hopeful pink lines only a matter of days earlier, I could almost sense the life being created inside of me. Now, all I felt was a dull ache that seemed to tangibly encapsulate the very concepts of death, loss, and emptiness. How was it possible for life to change so dramatically in such a short space of time?

"Normally at eight weeks, one would detect an image here," the doctor said, pointing at the monitor as she pushed severely against my belly with the scan wand. "But, this confirms a miscarriage. You won't require any further treatment as everything has gone." Her eyes stuck hard and fast to the screen as she delivered her ground-breaking statement with all the compassion of someone relaying the daily weather report. For a moment, I laid there taking in her words, my eyes piercing the side of her stone cold face, willing her to turn around and show me an ounce of sympathy. She never returned my gaze.

I jumped off the table and made a rather awkward dash for the door, rushing across the stark clinical corridor and into the bathroom just as the floodgates gave way. Standing with my back against the mirror so as to avoid looking into my own eyes, I sobbed uncontrollably, stifling the noise with the palms of my hands. The aching emptiness inside my womb seemed to deepen, sharpen, and blacken, as if in confirmation of the doctor's starkly stated findings. With it, came fierce waves of self-loathing unlike any I'd ever experienced before. I really was useless... it was all my fault that I'd lost my baby... I shouldn't have been so stupid as to drive on such an icy day. *What had I been thinking?* It had taken two years to finally see those cherished pink lines, and now my baby was gone. Just like that, because of me and my careless, stupid choices. *How could I possibly live with myself?*

Managing to avoid the mirror altogether, I pulled some tissue from the dispenser, dried my eyes, and made my way back out into the dark, heartless, senseless world, of which I officially no longer wanted any part. *But, what choice did I have?* For better or worse, I was here. Perhaps, if I could at least spend my life helping others, I could, maybe, somewhat, make up for my pitiful existence. I could counteract the extremely bad luck my mum had endured for ever having given birth to me.

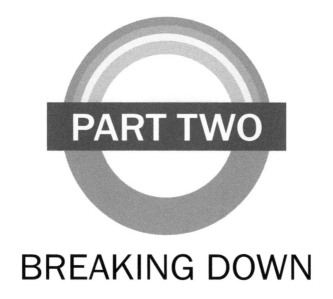

PART TWO

BREAKING DOWN

NINE

DYING TO LIVE

What on earth is life, and death, all about anyway?

Having Sandy as a manager increased my intrigue in all things spiritual even more, although I never dared say as much. She'd had such a deep faith that not even the biggest cynic could have denied themselves from wondering whether there had been anything in the glint she consistently had in her eye. So when she was suddenly taken, the shock only added to those thoughts, which still resonated with me from Katie's untimely death. We had been such a close team, and with Sandy at the helm it had felt as though we were invincible. It had been the first job, since the beginning of my mental health career, in which I'd actually felt valued and safe enough to stay for longer than a year. Sandy had been one of the main reasons for this. One day we had been laughing together in the team meeting, holed up in the central meeting room making the rest of the office wonder what we found so amusing when all we had to discuss was which of our clients were still homeless and how many we had on the waiting list. But with Sandy around there had always been a reason to giggle.

"I think this one's for you, Katie" she had said, as we looked at the details of the referral allocations. It was for a man who had a phobia of the colour pink. "Thanks very much!" I had retorted, laughing but taking slight offence at the allusion that I too had an aversion to such a girly colour.

"Well I can't see him, can I?" Sandy responded with a wry smile, "He won't be able to look at me!" My eyes focused on the pink lenses in her glasses, prescribed for her Meares-Irlen Syndrome. Feeling myself going flush in the cheeks, I graciously took the referral form and started scanning the detailed pages.

"Apart from that he has an issue with his extended family wanting him to leave, and I know how well you've dealt with a similar issue in the past. I also know that you will take his phobia seriously," Sandy had reassured. She always had a knack of making me feel good about myself.

Then one day, only three weeks later, she was gone.

It had been the bruises that had suddenly appeared which had alerted her to the fact that it must be more serious than the doctors had been saying. The tiredness hadn't just been due to stress and her migraines after all. She had taken herself away for her annual summer solstice treat; a camping trip up to the coast on her own. It was where she'd felt most at peace: in nature. It was as if on some deeper level she knew it was going to be her last holiday. The day after she returned she had collapsed and was taken to hospital, never to be discharged.

I stood in the doorway to her solitary hospital room; there had been too many people gathered around her bed to allow me to enter. Despite the presence of so many bodies, including her vicar, whom she had invited to help plan her woodland burial funeral, there was an overwhelming serenity filling the atmosphere. Sandy glanced over at me standing at the door. Seeing the tears welling in my eyes she smiled, kissed the tips of her fingers and blew me her last kiss. My body caught it in a breath-taking sensation of peace. It was as if she knew that everything was okay, even though there was so much panic happening all around her. What did she know that nobody else seemed to?

Having huge confusion over what I was missing in my life, and an even bigger sense of having no control over it, I threw myself into making sure life would be the best it could possibly be. What was there to lose? Clearly we didn't know when we were going to die and so we may as well live a life we wanted to live. We'd sell up and move to Spain. Living in the sun and having a stress-free life would make me happy. Training as a Scuba Dive Instructor was making my husband happy and I desperately wanted him to do what he loved too. I decided to train as a Personal Trainer, that way I could help make a living abroad. I was sure there would be overweight ex-pats that needed some help with losing the odd pound or two.

Whilst planning the move to Spain I continued to run, running had been something that had helped me to manage my depression; a regular boost of natural serotonin; it seemed to work much better than any anti-depressants. Now I had a reason to run more because I was training to work in the fitness field, but more importantly to me, I was also training to run the London marathon, in order to raise funds for Leukaemia Care in Sandy's memory. I had also always had a desire to write; it was kind of cathartic for me to splurge my innermost thoughts onto a clean blank sheet of a pretty notebook, a way of spring-cleaning out all of the rubbish that was clogging my head. And so I started a diary memoir; a day by day account of my gruelling training schedule alongside a step-by-step guide about moving, lock, stock and barrel, to another country. I woke up in the middle of the night and something, deep in the depths of my soul, urged me to go downstairs and switch on the computer. As the cursor flashed up on the screen my fingers took over, quicker than my brain could think. I wrote *"Run to the Sun"* at the top of the first page. That would be the title, I had no idea where that had come from, but I liked it.

It had been exciting, like I really was making a great escape. An escape from what, I wasn't really sure, but it felt good nonetheless. Travelling over on the ferry, and driving through France and then Spain, with nothing but the equity from our cottage sale in the bank, a plan to buy and convert a cave in which to live and create a future, had felt like true freedom and a dream come true. Could things get any better than this? Travelling along the open highways, watching the pine trees whizzing by as the sun streamed through the windows of the Ford Explorer, with my rock at my side and my trusty dog behind me, I felt like the luckiest woman alive. I breathed a sigh of relief, I would be happy from now on and because of that I'd make my husband happy too. God only knew, the poor man had suffered enough already from the impact of my depression and moodiness. This was a new start, and I'd make sure it was for the better. Any guilt I felt at leaving my parents behind was overtaken with a sense of pending resolution.

Cycling through the *campo* in the first few weeks, exploring my new territory, I had found myself on someone's farmland. I panicked. *What if the owner saw me and shouted? Or even worse shot at me?* I wouldn't be able to explain myself. I really had to have Spanish lessons to improve my ability to communicate. It was only right; after all I was living in their country so I should at least speak their language. A little old lady emerged from the doorway of the *cortijo*, all dressed in black, and started to make her way towards me. She was stooped over so much that it gave her a hunch in her back and made her stand even shorter than my almost dwarfish five feet. I froze. As she got closer I started to mumble;

"Lo siento, senora, lo siento," What was the word for "lost" again?

"Hola, senorita," she began, beaming her sun-wizened welcoming face up towards my, no doubt astounded, countenance. I breathed a huge sigh of relief; clearly she wasn't intending to have me shot. For the next half an hour I stood beaming back at her, flailing my arms in an attempt to express myself, nodding my head and making enthusiastic affirming noises in response to what I managed to figure out was her life story. When it was clear that she was making the most of having company she rarely had, I realised that if I didn't make my excuses and leave now, I could realistically be standing there until I too was wizened by the sun. Making my excuses, in the politest pigeon Spanish I could muster, I got back on my cycle and waved her adios. As I rode off over the hilltop, being careful to dodge the lizards that took their lives into their own hands by scurrying across the dry, pampas grass littered sandy paths, I smiled a contented smile. Down below a shepherd was herding his goats, the bells around their necks tinkling as they faithfully hopped across the rocky outcrop behind him. *What lovely simple people they are,* I thought to myself. *Finally we can have a stress-free life.*

"So how's it going then?" one of my close friends asked during a catch-up phone call a few months later. *I love the feel of the village, I love the people, I love the simple lifestyle, not to mention the weather, but I still feel an underlying unease with life. What the hell is wrong with me?* I thought.

"It's great," I replied. "I'm living the dream!"

Will I ever be satisfied? I mused, whilst lying on a sun lounger the next morning. I concluded that I must feel guilty for having such a sought-after lifestyle, I didn't deserve it after all. So I forced myself to sit at my desk, hidden away in the tiny office in our beautiful converted cave house, (the type of place where dreams come true), beads of sweat dripping from my brow as I worked on plans to build the activity holiday business. *Was my overheating due to the blazing midday sun outside, or was I desperately trying to fight off unwanted thoughts and feelings that kept attempting to enter my tired brain? Was I losing the battle with avoidance?*

Her touch had felt like electricity. It had only been an Indian head massage, all above board and in public, *but hadn't she lingered longer on mine than on anyone else?* And why had she been so keen for me to come back later that day, *could she feel this strange energy too?* It didn't make any sense at all. Neither had the "message" she'd given me after the therapy; *how could she get a message for me from spirit?* She was just a normal woman. A normal lesbian. *Why did that make me feel uncomfortable?* I didn't have a problem with gay people at all. I imagined her hands on my neck again, gently turning me to face her, leaning down until her deep green eyes bore into my very soul.

I couldn't possibly be feeling these feelings for this stranger; I must be mistaken. I was married to a good man and nothing like this had ever entered my head before, only when my husband had joked about me being gay with one of my friends. Had he sensed something about me that even I hadn't realised? Had his jokes been covering up a real fear of his that was somehow based in truth? I was so confused. She had intrigued me, not only because of her unusually mysterious green eyes that seemed to be uncomfortably magnetic, but because of her openness about all things spiritual. It seemed to come naturally to her and I wanted to know more. *It must just be that, an intrigue.* As hard as I tried to stop the feelings that surged within me, feelings I had never known before, the more confused and scared I became. *Was the Universe trying to wake me up to the reason why I had been so unhappy – had I been hiding from the fact that I was really gay? How could I keep hiding this now?* The whole situation felt completely out of my control, and yet strangely compelling. I desperately didn't want to do anything to hurt my husband. *But how could I hide from it now I felt the truth? How would I know if it was right to acknowledge how I was feeling?* I needed a sign to tell me what to do. What I meant by that I didn't quite know, but somehow I needed to be led. As I found myself driving behind the green-eyed lady one day a few weeks later I noticed the sticker displayed in the back window of her 4x4;

"Run to the Sun" it clearly said.

It was as if my soul had known about this encounter before it happened. The pull to follow my intrigue was unavoidably compelling. It was beyond logic, and the result was devastating, but had that devastation been a necessary step of my spiritual journey?

TEN

THE ULTIMATE GET OUT CLAUSE

*Being comfortably numb may be painless,
but being frozen for too long can lead
to frostbite and permanent loss.*

My life had never been so chaotic. It was like I was watching someone else's drama unfold, like one of those compelling soap operas that you can't help watching, a voyeur into someone else's crumbling life. Except that crumbling life wasn't someone else's, it was mine. The dam that I'd created to keep my unexpressed emotions at bay had suddenly burst. *How could I possibly resolve the chaos that facing my true feelings had caused?*

Maybe if I hid under the duvet for long enough everyone would forget about me and just get on with their lives. It sure as hell felt too scary to get out of bed. And the tears of shame and guilt about destroying my marriage that continuously flowed had made my face all red and puffy. It was impossible to go out in public and pretend that everything was okay looking like this. *What would they all say?* I dreaded to think what was being said about me anyway, and they wouldn't have been wrong, if they were saying I wasn't worthy of being alive. *I wasn't worthy of being alive*, this time I really meant it.

81

I'd failed. I'd let everyone down. Everything was out of control. I was out of control. *What on earth could I do about it now; surely there was only one solution?*

And then I was lying on the side of a dusty *carretera* in a little Spanish *pueblo* wearing only a white towelling dressing gown. I was vomiting and defecating, having become totally detached from my body after taking a massive overdose, the kind of overdose you take only if you really want to die. I really wanted to die. It didn't feel like me lying there, how could it possibly have come to this? I was always so strong, sensitive underneath obviously, but strong on the surface. I felt nothing. Numbness isn't painful. I did as I was instructed and got back into the passenger seat, staring vacantly out of the window until we arrived at the hospital. *Surely it couldn't be that serious? Couldn't they just leave me alone and allow me to disappear?* I didn't want to cause a fuss.

I slipped into the toilet and considered just locking the door and never coming out. I didn't care if I died in there, wrapped around the cistern on the cold tile floor, it's what I deserved and it would do everyone a favour. But I also knew that the green-eyed lady wouldn't let me, so I paced around and dutifully opened the lock when she knocked on the door to ask if I was okay in a shakily angry but caring voice. I tried to say I was sorry, but no words would come out.

I came-to, lying on a plastic sheet on a trolley. I had no idea how much time had passed. What felt like hoards of staff were around me trying to ram plastic tubing of various widths up my nose. It hurt; it really fucking hurt. They sounded panicked and I vaguely heard one of them say that it had been more than four hours. They were clearly angry with me. This wasn't the outcome I'd intended. In fact I hadn't intended any outcome at all. It had been an impulsive act, not a cry for help as I knew they'd suggest, (I'd said that about my patients before in any case), but an act of pure desperation – *what was life all about when you'd completely messed it up and couldn't work out a resolution?*

For moments during the waves of semi-consciousness my feelings returned, those familiar feelings of guilt I knew only too well. I was right, my mum should never have had me. It would have saved her a lifetime of anguish, my husband the pain I had caused him, and everyone connected to me now the inconvenience of this situation. There weren't any words to describe how I felt. You don't learn this kind of vocabulary or how to deal with these situations at school, why would you need to? *Things like this don't happen in real life.* Numbness was the only option. It should be me looking after me, not me being the patient.

I finally came-round properly in a bed with metal sides. I looked across the room, all full of beeping machines, at the beds opposite and saw two other people with tubes coming out of their noses, it was only then that I remembered I had one too. It hurt to swallow; it must have scratched my throat as it went down into my stomach in an attempt to pump out the toxins I had ingested. The young man opposite suddenly sat up and pulled out his tube, a long bloody worm of plastic wriggling out of a black hole in his tormented face. I cringed.

My heart went out to the staff that rushed to sort him out, I understood the anxiety he must have been causing them. Only now I was causing that same anxiety too. Anxiety that I used to feel when dealing with the patients on the ward where I worked, trying to understand what made people get into such a state that made them want to hurt themselves, so that I could help them and prevent it. Oh the irony. I noticed that the heart monitor next to the bed of the young man was displaying a pretty steady rhythm, like smooth humps on the back of a multi-humped camel. Mine, on the other hand, was the shape of erratic mountain peaks, like nasty crevices beneath rocky outcrops. I suddenly felt like a climber, small and insignificant clinging to a vast rock face, frozen in fear, petrified of falling. *Maybe I did want to live after all?*

A few staff nurses came over to my bed and, unlocking the brakes, began wheeling me over closer to the observation window where they all sat, like visitors to a zoo observing the animals through the protective glass. If they ensured enough distance, they couldn't be affected. I noticed that I was feeling frightened. I felt completely alone in a foreign country and everything was a total mess. It wasn't a nice feeling and I'd rather go back to feeling nothing at all. They still seemed to be angry with me, and kept asking me what I'd taken. I'd told them everything, and yet still they questioned, as if I was lying or not telling the whole story. They frequently returned and clumsily took more blood and changed over the bags hanging from the metal saline drip stand by the side of me, as if they may even have been trying to cause me more pain. I was aware that I was a costly inconvenience; I'd heard that said about people like me before too. I had no idea how long I'd been there, how many bags of saline solution had gone through me and back out into a bag connected to me by yet another tube "down below". I had never known so much shame and degradation. And it was all self-inflicted.

Until that moment I had been mute, the only communication coming from my pleading eyes and half-smile. Apologetic and pathetic. I don't really know how it happened, but when the Psychiatrist came into the ward to talk to me, I felt his warmth and suddenly Spanish was flowing from my mouth as if I'd spoken it my whole life. I wanted him to know everything, just like my headmistress on that morning fifteen years previously; I needed him to understand what had brought me to this horrific moment.

I told him everything. About Mum's suicide attempt and how she had been unwell since I was born, about how I got married because I wanted to make everything okay and didn't even realise I was gay. How I blamed myself for having a miscarriage. How I moved to Spain to make a better life and fell in love with a woman, and how terribly guilty I felt about the whole situation. I also told him that I was sorry for causing such a fuss and that I felt very stupid: "*Estupida*". And then he told me that they'd found *"Polvo de Angel"* in my system: Angel dust. *What is that?* I wondered, and *how on earth had they found traces of it in me?* And then it all started to make sense.

I had been away on a weekend break in Granada a few weeks previously, I told him, and recalled a night where I'd had a very strange experience. I had felt very unsteady on returning to my hotel room and, as far as I was aware, passed out until about twelve hours later. The next morning I had been told that I hadn't passed out at all, but had been acting out-of-character, and my eyes had been rolling and bloodshot. I had laughed it off as too much alcohol, although I hadn't drunk a huge amount and had encountered no hangover, which with hindsight seemed very odd indeed. I had thought no more about it at the time.

The realisation hit me like a slap in the face. I remembered the barman at the last bar pouring the drinks at the back of the counter, not on the bar as is customary in Spain. *I had been spiked.* A strange mixture of relief and disbelief washed over me. This gave me an excuse. I could blame the drugging for my erratic behaviour, and yet the deed was still done and the consequences still the same. I noticed the shift in how the staff nurses treated me from that moment on, suddenly empathy oozing from them and into my heart, and it gave me the strength to smile a wider smile and make my apologies more evident. I wished I could stay there, it felt safe, like a bubble of calm in a chaotic world that was completely alien to me. But I had created that alien world, and so back out into it, I had no choice, but to go.

The return was excruciating. I realised, that in trying my utmost to avoid hurting anyone else, by attempting the ultimate escape, I had achieved exactly what I had been trying to avoid. I had affected those around me in the same way my mum had affected me with her own suicide attempt. I felt consumed with guilt and concluded that I'd never be able to forgive myself. That I had to try to make it up to the people, about whom I cared, by forgetting my own feelings again and focusing on them. How could I be so selfish now as to think about my own needs? Deep down, despite everything, I still knew that I wasn't a bad person, despite what I imagined everyone in the village was saying about me, hurting anyone other than myself had never even crossed my mind, although I could see why it looked that way. *Maybe they were right and I really was bad?* I felt confused and empty. Too afraid to let my feelings in, in case they took over again and made things even worse, if that were at all possible. And so I shut down, it was easier than admitting how vulnerable I felt. Too weak to admit I had made a mistake. Admitting that would make me weak. If I just got on with life for everyone else's sake that was the best I could manage. And so nothing was mentioned and the pattern of repressed emotions resumed. I was frozen, and it was going to take something pretty epic to thaw me out.

ELEVEN

GETTING NAKED WITH YOURSELF

*"One of the bravest things you can
do in life is to own your own story."*

BRENE BROWN

I had never known I was capable of feeling, let alone expressing, so much anger. As the cutting words left my lips they shocked me; *was that really me shouting?* I had always been so meek and mild. I was scaring myself. I had lost control of my emotions and I had no idea how I was going to regain it. It was far easier to blame everyone around me for my lack of happiness than to face the fact that I felt completely and utterly lost. Who was I really angry at? Looking back, it would have been a safe bet to say "Myself".

As the plane taxied along the hazy runway I breathed a sigh of relief. The sigh, however, was incongruous to the volcano of panic that was rising inside. Where on earth would I start with recreating a life back in the UK now I had lost everything? How would I meet anyone or get back on the housing ladder? I desperately wanted the security of a loving relationship, but I knew nothing about the gay scene, and the thought of being in it frightened me to death. *Was I doing the right thing or had I made a huge mistake? Maybe it would have been easier to deny my feelings and have held on to the security I had so recklessly thrown away? How would I ever know if I had done the right thing by facing my sexuality?* I needed another sign.

The bubbly, blonde curly-haired girl sitting next to me ordered a whisky and coke from the flight attendant as he pushed the refreshment trolley along the aisle. In fact she ordered two. It was only then I noticed how giggly and tactile she was being with the girl sitting on her other side. She turned to me and asked if I'd like her to order anything for me. "I know it's a bit early for a drink", she laughed, "but we're celebrating; we're on honeymoon."

"Oh how lovely!" I exclaimed, unable to hide the surprised look that must have appeared on my face. They were pretty girls, and they seemed really normal. *Maybe it was possible for me to meet someone in everyday life after all?* And then I felt bad. *Why had I thought that wasn't the case? Had I been unwittingly perpetuating my own stigma?* Raising my own plastic glass to theirs, I breathed a genuine sigh of relief. I was on the right path.

So all I needed to do was get myself another job, find a partner, and then I'd finally be happy. It was quite simple really. At least I still had Vinnie to confide in, now I understood why Mum had been so close to Jill. Thinking of him caged away in the hold of the plane made the guilt resurface once again, I was getting used to the palpitations in my chest and waves of nausea that seemed to be an everyday occurrence at the moment; my new "normality" was a world away from that of the monotony of the life I lived in my pre-Spain, Norfolk cottage. It must still be the effects of the Angel Dust, I reassured myself; they had said it would stay in my system for at least six months.

Getting back to work did prove to be simple. In no time I was again working for the mental health charity that I had left only two years previously. It was like I'd never even been away, and it felt like returning to the family fold; yet I had returned a completely different person. I couldn't let on how much personal turmoil those two years had contained; *how could I possibly support people with mental health problems when my own was in such a mess?* But it wasn't anymore; I was back on familiar ground. I had survived. *Everything would be fine. I was fine.* I'd wear my fake smile as I had done previously and nobody would know a thing.

Running kept me afloat again. Every time unwelcomed emotions surfaced, I managed to silence them with enforced adrenalin. And finding a girlfriend hadn't been as hard as I'd imagined. I had what I had been looking for; a new job and the promise of a "happy-ever-after" relationship; but the happiness that it was supposed to bring was still evasive. *Did I deserve to be happy, after being so ungrateful for life? I was a walking disaster – who was I anyway?* I went to a poetry workshop in an attempt to rekindle my writing;

Who Am I?
I am Katie. I am a Mottram, a ****, no longer either.
I am a broken oar; futile in a relentless rapid.

I am a weeping Willow, suffocating in the shadows of vast
  Oaks.
I am a chrysalis hanging by a thread, screaming for freedom.
Who Am I?
I am a blood-stained kitchen knife in a hospital corridor,
Reflecting the pallor of a head held between trembling knees,
the stench of sterilisation.
I refuse to be an ostrich. I am a palpitation, a lack of motivation,
A spinning top refusing to stop; inherited suicidal tendencies.
I am a fake smile. "I am fine".
I am a pair of weighing scales, I am soaring on a thermal,
Wind in my ears and warmth on my wings...and then I am
  lead, metallic and hollow.
I am an extended ride on the big dipper, "Stop, I want to get off!"
I am interdisciplinary, because it's easier, I am ambiguity.
Who Am I?
I am that fake smile hiding inside a white dress; an expectation,
I am making everything better. "I am fine".
I am an oven for a bun, I am someone – and then-
I am not a mum.
I am wrapped around a tree trunk with shattered bodywork.
I am smashed, I am strong, I am a Portland vase bleeding
  from every pore,
until I'm empty.
Who Am I?
I run, and run, and run, and run... "I am fine".
I am a sponge for all your woes, I am dripping with your tears,
projected traumas and unrequited desires.

I am a crumbling wall, a dirge.

I am a problem, a solution, a shield,

a hypocrite, a fraud, logical, illogical, contrary.

Who Am I?

I am a spirit level, kinetic, nutritious, going somewhere...
   "I am fine".

I am bleached, I am tanned, a glowing chasm.

I am safe hiding in my cave, I am denial.

I am ripping off the white dress, fuck the expectations!

I am a butterfly.

Who Am I?

I am an incomplete puzzle, destroyer, traitor, destroyed.
   "I am fine".

I am Neanderthal, a foetus in a puddle of infinite tears.

I am numb, I am orgasmic, I CAN feel.

I am not safe hiding in my cave.

I am a masochist, obliterated, a failure.

Who Am I?

I am vomit, I am intubated, an exhibition for curious eyes.

I am "loca". "I am fine".

I am a nightmare, but I am not dreaming.

I am waiting to be shot by a star.

I am here, I am now, and I am proud..."I will be fine".

Who Am I?

The words had flowed as if through my own hand but from somewhere beyond my brain again. *Did I really feel like this?* I hadn't even realised. *Who the fuck was I, and how was I supposed to find out?*

These feelings of loneliness weren't what I'd envisaged from a new relationship full of promise.

"You're pathetic" she said, and I sobbed with the longing for someone to love me for whom I was. *But how could anyone love me when I didn't really know who I was?* I was sensitive, I couldn't help that. Maybe that wasn't how I should be and I really was pathetic. I had to toughen up, to stop myself from getting even more hurt. Enough was enough.

Rosy was a new referral. She had been given to me to assess due to her locality, but I already sensed that I would be able to empathise with her situation. I think the team knew that too, although nobody had said anything. My heart pounded as I knocked on the door to her dingy flat. The concrete stairwell smelled of stale urine and I could see why living here would have a negative effect on anyone's mental wellbeing, before even considering everything else this young lady had gone through. I knew the outline of her story; I was here now to find out what she wanted me to do to help her move on from it.

The door opened a crack and a pair of petrified eyes peered at me through the skinny slit that the hefty security chain allowed. I flashed her my most welcoming smile and held up my identity badge;

"Hi, I'm Katie," I offered.

"Oh sorry," she replied, shakily, "I've been getting so much hassle from the guy on the next floor, I thought you might be him."

She ushered me in, locking the door again behind me. I thought she looked harmless enough, but I instinctively positioned myself on the chair closest to the only other evident escape route.

"I completely understand, it's best to be cautious when you're in such an unknown environment," I reassured, thinking that was maybe something that I could add to her case for alternative accommodation.

"Obviously I'm here to discuss the referral from your social worker, and to see how we may be able to help you. I've got an assessment form to go through, but I know it's a lot to ask to expect you to talk about everything the first time you meet me, so please only talk about as much as you feel comfortable."

Two and a half hours later, Rosy had poured out much more detail than I'd had from her very matter-of-fact referral. I knew that she had been released from hospital only a couple of weeks previously, having split from her husband just before being sectioned. She had been placed in this temporary flat straight from the ward, having had nowhere else to go. She had tried to cope with the changes on her own, too ashamed to admit that her finances, on top of her emotions, were in a complete mess. She told me that she felt like she was sinking again, and was petrified that she'd end up dead like her mum. She told me the doctor had told her that her mum's disorder was likely to be hereditary, and as much as she had fought with him about that at the time, she was now wondering if he was right. I had told her categorically that, the fact that she'd had such an emotional response to everything she'd been holding back from expressing, didn't mean that she had a "disorder"; it actually meant that she was human. I had spoken to her from my heart, reassuring her that anyone who had gone through as much as her would have had to break down at some point, and that it was nothing, of which to be ashamed. Only a robot could experience the suicide of their mother, the unfulfilled longing of a child lost through miscarriage and subsequent marriage breakdown, and carry on as if everything was okay. I had suggested that her mother's death hadn't been about her, it was due to unresolved issues her mum had been carrying, that had not been her responsibility, or over which she had any control. I advised her that the strongest thing she could do would be to finally stop fighting and to deal with her deep-rooted and overriding feelings of guilt she told me she felt, that were serving nobody and destroying everything.

"I really must get going", I exclaimed, suddenly realising the time along with the fact that I had actually achieved to complete very little of my official form. As much as I would have loved to stay and talk to Rosy for the rest of the afternoon, I had to get to another appointment.

"I'm so sorry I've kept you so long and you've not even done what you needed to", she apologised profusely.

"Not at all", I quickly replied, "I'm really glad you felt able to tell me so much, I hope it has helped".

"I don't quite know why I told you everything I did, it usually takes me ages to open up to anyone" Rosy blushed.

We held a gaze of mutual respect and understanding. I knew exactly why she had found it so easy to open up to me.

As I drove home that evening my words of advice rang in my own ears. *The strongest thing you could do would be to stop fighting and deal with your deep-rooted and overriding feelings.* I knew it was time to stop running. I needed to talk about everything, lay everything bare and finally get naked with myself. I felt quite sick all of a sudden.

When I arrived home I wrote a card to mark the end of yet another failed relationship. "You can't set sail with your anchor still attached" my hand wrote, although I had no idea where the words had come from, or what they even meant. *Who said that, and what did it mean? Were the words really meant for me?*

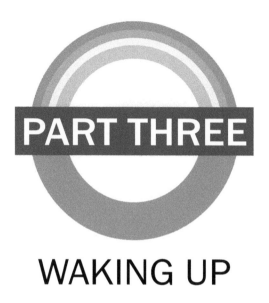

PART THREE

WAKING UP

TWELVE

FROM BREAKDOWN
TO BREAKTHROUGH

"All great changes are preceded by chaos."

DEEPAK CHOPRA

My body had finally forced me to stop running, the pain in my left knee was excruciating. Looking back I guess my body had had to speak to me as I wasn't listening to my emotional state crying-out for attention. Frustrated at my inability to exercise and worried that I would pile on weight and feel even worse about myself, I decided to start yoga again. Something about the gentle practice and nurturing, quiet confidence of my teacher, Lou, spoke to that part of me, deep inside, that had been searching for "something" for as long as I could remember. Yoga reassured me that it was okay to be searching, and that my yearning for something more, something different from the Western world around me, wasn't quite as crazy as I had been led to believe. The escape from external chaos during savasana was intriguing, and I craved it more and more. Lou, who ran Yoga Happy in Norwich, had just embarked on a training course entitled "Yoga for the Mind", studying the impact of yoga on depression. When she made an appeal for case studies during a class one evening, something made me volunteer, although the thought of opening myself up in this way to someone so seemingly confident petrified me.

I started to practice meditation on my own, to "BE with myself" for the first time ever, and it was hard work. *How could sitting still be so demanding?* It took some practice, but I finally got to the point where I could sit without fidgeting, wondering what to have for dinner, or peeping to see if anyone was laughing at me for at least ten minutes at a time. Eventually, the benefits were outweighing my fears about what anyone thought of me. And then something profound happened.

On this particular day I was feeling pretty exasperated with work; frustrated at what I still considered to be overly-imposed inhumane boundaries, and feeling uninspired by a soulless system which liked labelling people seemingly to an inch of their lives. I felt like a fraud, *how was I any different to these people I was discussing for referral when I'd spent so long feeling emotionally unstable and confused?*

Sitting in the middle of my bed that evening I said silently to myself , *"So what the hell is mental illness all about anyway?"* It hadn't been an intentional question, (well, there had been nobody to whom a question could be addressed), but merely an off-loading of my frustration into the ether. Looking back, it had been complete surrender. I had reached a point when I knew I couldn't pretend to have all of the answers anymore; I was desperate for some kind of insight, some kind of proof of that, which I had always felt to be true; that there was more to life than trudging along, making out that I was happy to live with this nagging sense of having something missing inside, when actually I wasn't at all. Thinking nothing of this momentous shift in my internal defences, I began a meditation and, for the first time ever, was able to clear my mind of all thoughts. It was as if the rail track had been cleared, and I wasn't prepared for the train that was about to come hurtling along at full speed, a real-life Starlight Express, bursting with a freight of information direct from the Universe.

I focused on my breath. As usual, I could feel my heart rate, previously raised by my agitated mood, slow down as my muscles relaxed and my awareness of the bed beneath my backside disappeared. I could hear the birds gently singing outside the bedroom window, all chirpy in the emerging spring air; Oh to be that stress-free I thought. And then there was nothing. I'd never experienced thinking "nothing" before. It was really quite odd, but very liberating at the same time. I watched for my thoughts as if I was watching for a mouse emerging from a dark hole in a skirting board. I had started to read *The Power of Now* by Eckhart Tolle, and this had been his advice. At first some thoughts tried to escape through the hole, but when I gently pushed them back they disappeared altogether. When I'd read about this stuff before I had thought it sounded like nonsense, how on earth was it possible not to think? I was constantly chatting away and arguing with myself in my head. But my thoughts had stopped coming; and there I found myself. Me. The very thing I had felt was missing, the thing that had evaded me for so many years; it hadn't been a "thing" at all, but my very self! I became aware of my soul watching for my thoughts. I became aware of my soul watching me, sitting on my bed, and it spoke to me with such clarity;

"You are a vehicle to bring about spiritual awareness; you will help to develop an easily comprehensible framework about spiritual crisis to reduce the stigma of mental illness and to increase the understanding of us as spiritual beings within modern society. Mental illness will be redefined in terms of spirituality."

Who said that? My thoughts were back. I opened my eyes to see if there was someone who had spoken to me. I was still alone. But I knew the words I'd heard – well, more like "felt" – dropped into my consciousness; it was hard to define. And I knew these words were more real than the bed on which my backside was now becoming numb. My soul, the "real" me, had been waiting to communicate with me for thirty-six years. I hadn't been ready before. But now I knew, I wasn't bloody mad – Western society was! To my utter amazement, in that split moment my question about the reality of mental illness had been answered so clearly and without any doubt, that everything I had ever contemplated about my existence in the world made complete sense; more sense than I had ever dreamed it was possible to know. I laughed out loud to myself! I had been desperately searching for answers to the meaning of life, to what it was all about, outside of myself for so long, and actually, all I'd needed to do was look within; all of those weird spiritual teachings were bloody true! After years of searching for my life purpose it had been handed to me on a plate, quite literally from the Universe straight into my head, like a light bulb suddenly being switched on in a dark, deep cave of confusion. In that moment I had experienced a profound awareness of my soul, my core essence, and what shocked me the most was that I actually liked my soul! I had awoken from being someone who felt completely helpless and insignificant in the world, to having an innate knowledge that I had the potential to be anyone I wanted to be, because every human being is equal, (hierarchy was just a futile construct), and that I could achieve anything, upon which I set my heart. I felt awash with an inexplicable sense of awe and excitement for life, and knew I was completely protected in what can only be described as a Universal bubble of unconditional love. Any resentment I had been harbouring, all fear for the future, had completely disappeared. Death no longer scared me, my soul was eternal, and so I was free to enjoy life – I was free to be brave and not worry about what anyone thought of me anymore – but most importantly of all, I was able to forgive myself for every mistake that had gone before. It was the past and I was free to make my future the best it could possibly be.

I grabbed a pad of paper and a pen and proceeded to write three whole sides of A4. When I looked down I saw that it was a theory about mental distress; a theory I had known nothing about an hour before! It was as if something beyond my head was controlling the pen in my hand. Here I was experiencing the biggest paradox of life, and I only knew that, as the explanation was written before my eyes. I had spent a long time on the brink of emotional crisis, grappling to find answers, but now I knew that my crisis had been part of the process – a "spiritual emergence". I had been on the brink of true sanity!

My message from the Universe, on the page in front of me, told me everything I needed to know; that mental distress is a portal into self-actualisation, providing a gateway into inner-consciousness, to the core of our being, and is only labelled as an "illness" because of how we have been conditioned to understand it within Western culture.

This is exactly why a spiritual emergence becomes so distressing, because society tells us that what we are experiencing is wrong; that is the real insanity! *How bloody ironic!* The message continued. If mental distress and our natural "sixth sense" can be accepted as part of natural human development, and we learn to accept them as our normality as opposed to "abnormal", they consequently become less scary and do not create such an adverse reaction within us. Ultimately we are all spiritual beings pretending not to be, and by denying ourselves our true nature, somewhere deep down we sense something isn't right. Therefore we try to fill this void by accumulating more and more materialistically or experientially, whereas all this does is push us further away from self-discovery. When people who begin to experience extreme emotions are diagnosed as mentally ill, it can block their spiritual evolution as they become afraid of their feelings (if they haven't already been suppressed with medication), which can exacerbate the symptoms.. The Ego acts as a kind of protector against perceived fear, but it is actually fooling us as these are unfounded fears, so we need to push beyond the Ego barrier in order to discover that there really was nothing to fear in the first place. When we function only at an Ego level we are shut down from our true emotions and function robotically; here we look for fleeting happiness which we seek in the material world or through connections with other people. True happiness can never be found here, it can only be found within. The consequence of continuing to live in this disconnected robotic mode would eventually mean that we destroy ourselves and the human race. Facing our perceived fears is the only way to extinguish them; and to be free to evolve.

On one level I knew that my level of consciousness had expanded and that the message I had been given was the absolute truth; *but how could this be happening?* I felt awash with a deep clarity and relief. Every part of my life up to this point had been meant to happen to bring me to here. For the first time ever I felt huge gratitude for all of the difficult times, because I now knew that they had happened to wake me up. *Synchronicity – this was my calling.* What did Synchronicity mean? I'd never heard that word before! *This was bloody weird!* At the same time as thinking it was weird, at a deeper level I knew in my heart that my life purpose was to highlight that the mental health system is antiquated, and that it's time we stop pretending we're robots in a naturally spiritual world. *That was why I was here.* My soul had chosen my life experience in order to be part of an evolutionary shift. All of that clairvoyance crap that Mum had been going on about for years was actually true! She wasn't mad at all; she had just broken down with the frustration at being unable to speak her truth. My poor mum. How strong she really was to have held this secret for so many years. I now felt her truth too; and it was so amazing and affirming, and yet I had disbelieved her and played a part in getting her hospitalised. No wonder she had felt so helpless and angry. But it was fine, and this time not in a "Fucked-up, Insecure, Neurotic and Emotional" way, but it really *would* be fine – my soul just *knew* it! I could make it up to her now, finally. I would talk to Mum about my experience, and apologise for disbelieving her experiences for so many years.

Okay, so now I had been given a clear message and told that I was to deliver this message on behalf of the Universe. I was excited beyond belief. *Holy Shit! How the hell was I going to relay this message and not get sectioned? Why me, of all people? Who was I and what did I know about re-evaluating the conceptual framework around mental illness or achieving universal peace?* But I knew that this was exactly why the information had come to me; the fact that I wasn't anyone special. That was the point entirely; this had nothing to do with social stature or intelligence. I had been given this message to prove that anybody can access the psychic realm and see a universal truth, that we are all exactly the same. *The Universe obviously knows that I'm a stubborn so-and-so, that once I get my mind set on something I don't give up; Bugger, why couldn't I be more flimsy?!* Now I really had gone and let myself in for it; I knew this was big, and it wasn't going to go away.

I felt euphoric. I felt like shouting from the rooftops that I had found the meaning of life and that it was all going to be okay, we just all needed to look within and love each other! I never thought I'd sound like such a hippy! But then my logical, "professional" brain kicked-in and brought me tumbling back to earth with a bump. I had worked in the mental health field for long enough to know the academic theory, and my "logical" thoughts slapped me around the face with the sheer panic that I was psychotic. What had happened was too real for even my doubting brain to convince me that I had gone mad, but I knew that if I talked openly about my experience and new beliefs that I would be considered to be delusional. *What on earth was I going to do?* This was the most wonderful experience of my life and yet I was unable to talk about it; all that did was further convince me that things needed to change. *How many other people had experienced this, been sectioned and medicated due to a very real spiritual experience, or conversely, been driven crazy by the inability to express themselves for fear of being seen as mad?*

The next three days only served to further convince me that I had to do something, I got more and more proof that what was happening to me, although evading logic completely, was indeed very real. I had never had so much energy. Cycling effortlessly to a training day the next morning I watched a bird flying overhead. An overpowering sense of bliss washed over me as I experienced for a moment actually "being" that bird, soaring and free, able to see my surroundings from its higher perspective, and my eyes filled with tears of happiness. I knew that I was intricately connected to the magical world around me. Ordinarily, attending a training event such as this with colleagues who were mostly more academically experienced than me would have filled me with anxiety and a sense of inferiority, but today I felt their equal. Having never studied the Social Care Law that was being discussed, it came as a bit of a shock when I realised I knew everything that was being spoken about. *But how could I possibly know something that I'd never studied before?* Raising my hand to answer a question that nobody else appeared to have the confidence to answer, I was aware that my former, very insecure, shy self was being supported by my Higher Self, which had access to the infinite information from universal consciousness. I felt a paradox of emotions all rolled into one; insurmountable joy and absolute terror at what was happening to me. I knew, without a shadow of a doubt, that what I was experiencing was very special and real, and yet at the same time my brain would not let me believe it. *What if I had Bi-polar disorder?*

What if I had really gone mad and if I spoke out risked following in my mum's footsteps faced with a lifetime of heavy drugs and having to forget all about what had happened? What if these really were the ramblings of an unstable mind?

Cycling home I decided that I had no choice. It was an arduous task but deep down I knew that the real insanity would be for me to ignore such an important task and deny myself my own truth for fear of speaking out, because all that would achieve would be to drive me insane. *Oh the irony!* What kind of hypocrite would I be if I were to tell everyone that they didn't need to be scared, that this kind of stuff is actually normal, if I was too afraid to put my head above the parapet and risk being shot at? I needed another sign that I had to speak out.

Arriving home I turned on the laptop. A quote on *Facebook* grabbed my attention:

"You may be 38 years old, as I happen to be. And one day, some great opportunity stands before you and calls you to stand up for some great principle, some great issue, some great cause. And you refuse to do it because you are afraid. You refuse to do it because you want to live longer. You're afraid that you will lose your job, or you are afraid that you will be criticized, or that you will lose your popularity, or you're afraid that somebody will stab you, or shoot at you or bomb your house; so you refuse to take the stand. Well, you

may go on and live until you are 90, but you're just as dead at 38 as you would be at 90. And the cessation of breathing in your life is but the belated announcement of an earlier death of the spirit."

DR MARTIN LUTHER KING JR.

And there it was; my message. Direct from Martin Luther King. At least I had two years to build up the confidence! I knew that I needed to do some research. I needed to find evidence that what I needed to say wasn't madness. I needed to find other people who had experienced similar things; *surely I couldn't be the only one?* A Google search led me to Professor Chris Cook. He was a Psychiatrist but also a lecturer in Spirituality, Theology and Health; if anyone was going to understand this stuff then it was likely to be him. My gut told me to email him, and so before I had time to talk myself out of it I typed an anonymous message explaining all about my experience and the theory I had channelled. He was far enough away and there was no way he'd know who I was if he thought I was completely bonkers; I was safe. Still my heart pounded as I pressed "send".

It had been a risk but one, it turned out, to be well worth taking.

THIRTEEN

JOINING PIECES OF THE PUZZLE

"The inspiration you seek is already within you.
Be silent, and listen."

RUMI

A new message flashed up in my inbox. I could see that it had come from Durham University: Professor Cook had replied. I hesitated as the cursor hovered over "open"; what if he suggested I go and get a mental health assessment and totally negated my experience? I fully expected that this would be the case. My heart pounded in my chest and nausea swept over me once again; if only I could find someone who understood I knew would be on the right road to achieving the task I had been given through my message. Reading the content of the email made me wish that this man wasn't so far away after all! It was wonderfully supportive and, although admitting that he couldn't validate my experience as it was so subjective, he assured me that saying such things did not make me sectionable. I wanted to hug him! Little did this virtual, open-minded professional stranger, know that he had helped me over my first and biggest hurdle; he had provided me with the strength I needed to believe in my truth. For the first time in my life I felt like I actually knew myself, and could start to believe that I did really did have something to offer the world after all.

I had every faith that everything would work out in the end, but absolutely no idea about how I would get there, or in fact, where "there" even was. There was a huge chasm between where I was, and where I knew I needed to get. All I knew was that I had to remain quiet and be careful who I told, whilst I researched more and settled into my experience. Being someone who found it difficult to keep my opinions to myself at the best of times, this would prove an almighty task! If only I could find an outlet for this information that was so alien, and yet bubbling away inside of me with such clarity and passion to be released. I needed to find other people who understood, *surely there must be others?* I knew that there was a danger in keeping my new beliefs to myself, (the message I channelled had told me such), but I also knew that people would be quick to judge if I spoke too openly about them – my experience with Mum and through work was evidence enough of that. My thoughts turned to Mum again. I realised just how strong she had been to have survived for all of these years, keeping something so profound and intrinsic to herself, a virtual secret; there was no bloody wonder it had sent her round the twist! I had never had the understanding to view her situation with such compassion before, and now I felt compelled to spread the message about how destructive it is that we view spiritual experiences as "abnormal" within Western society. Things needed to change not only for the sake of my mum, but for the hundreds and thousands of people who already had, or were at risk of, being labelled as mad when they weren't at all. I felt completely blessed. Most people who have deep spiritual experiences don't have a framework within which to understand them; but the Universe had provided me with an understanding which I would be able to relay to others, who were also "waking up" to their spirituality and falling foul of a mental health system that was pathologising them for doing so. The whole system was insane – not the people in it! *Maybe I could write a book?* That way I could pass on any messages I wanted to, and maintain my anonymity. *But why was I so scared of people knowing who I was when the message I wanted to give was that this weird stuff needs to be normalised?* I was being a hypocrite and my confidence needed some work. If I was going to do it, I'd have to be brave. The thought made me want to throw up instantly.

Marie had been a colleague for years, I trusted her and I also knew that her husband was a Buddhist, and so she was open-minded about spirituality. Before I'd even given it a second thought, I heard the words spilling out of my mouth. "I know it sounds crazy, Marie, but I had access to Universal consciousness and I just know that the information I got is true".

"What you describe sounds exactly like something a friend of mine has written a book about", Marie replied, completely stony-faced. *How hadn't I known about this before?* I wondered, *do you mean to say that this is common knowledge and yet, even working in the mental health system, we haven't been made aware of it?* Astounded, I bombarded Marie with an inquisition to rival the Spanish. I was now equipped with the knowledge of not only another individual who understood the experience of waking up to another level of consciousness, but a whole network of individuals who had united in their experiences in order to spread this vital information; *The UK Spiritual Crisis Network*. This was apparently something Marie's friend Catherine had developed in order to support those in spiritual crisis to understand what they were going through. It not only existed in the UK; there was also a network in America. Tears of relief blurred my vision as I scanned the words on their website (www.spiritualcrisisnetwork.org.uk) later that evening:

From Breakdown to Breakthrough; Promoting understanding and support for those going through profound personal transformation.

"Spiritual crisis (often called Spiritual Emergency, Emergence, Awakening or psycho-spiritual crisis), is a turbulent period of spiritual opening and transformation.

We recognise that spiritual crisis and mental health difficulties often overlap.

Yes! It really was true, I wasn't mad at all! Tears continued to flow freely as I excitedly emailed the information contact.

I had to get to know these people, I was supposed to be involved with what they were doing – it was that synchronicity thing in action.

I could feel my emotions getting out of control again. All of this had been hugely overwhelming for my little brain, and I was finding it hard not to swing between total rapture that something so profound and amazing was happening to me, and feeling completely swamped by the pressure I was putting on myself to get on with being a "vehicle" to help relay this important message. *People had to know! People were suffering unnecessarily and it had to stop.* I knew speaking in this way made me sound like I had bi-polar disorder and ideas of grandiosity to my work colleagues; I knew that because I'd spoken about people in that way before. But now I knew how it felt to have this knowledge burning away inside, and I knew for a fact it wasn't any kind of "disorder".

My invitation to the Mindspan course being delivered by my new friend, Linda, couldn't have come at a better time. Everything Linda said that day spoke to me at a profound level. Before my experience I would have heard the teachings of the Mindspan techniques as sound psychological advice, and yet now I knew just how vital they were to living, not only a fulfilled life, but a life that was true to your soul purpose. The day left me feeling completely empowered. I had been given the kick I needed to embrace some facts with the seriousness it warranted; my thoughts and self-belief really were the things that were controlling my destiny, and by believing myself to be small and incapable of big things, I was the only one holding myself back. I finally realised that it was okay to admit that everything wasn't okay, that I still had deep-rooted emotional issues that I needed to resolve. It wasn't weak to admit this, it was actually the bravest thing I could do. Despite my epiphany, I had so many limiting beliefs that would seep into my thoughts, including the belief that I wasn't good enough and could never achieve anything significant, because I wasn't significant myself. But those beliefs didn't need to be true, if I no longer chose to believe them. Mindspan had taught me that my life was all about choices, and in a day it had confirmed that I could choose not to be afraid of failure. It had made the very intangible Universal information that I had felt so profoundly, make complete logical sense; *the pieces of the puzzle were finally coming together!*

Chris was also on the Mindspan course. She had been a work colleague, of whom I had initially been a bit wary. She was self-assured and said that she communicated with Angels and had done since childhood. I had been intrigued, even if slightly pessimistic. However, since my awakening experience, Chris had been someone, to whom I had grown increasingly close. I knew that I could say anything to her that may sound quite bizarre to most people, and she wouldn't bat an eyelid; in fact, she'd more than likely laugh at me for doubting myself. I confided in my "Angel Lady" friend one day, admitting to her that I knew I had some deep-rooted feelings of guilt that were holding me back, but I couldn't work out where they were coming from.

"We'll do a regression," Chris announced in her usual matter-of-fact, no messing about way.

And so we did. I sat on her couch whilst she talked me back, through a deep meditation, to the time my soul knew that I was "stuck". Where I ended up shocked my conscious mind, it had not been the thing I was expecting to surface. I had always been aware that I was carrying guilt about causing my mum's post natal depression through being born, and guilt at destroying my marriage through not realising I was gay. But I thought that I had let that go now as I knew that I didn't need to reprimand myself for hurt I hadn't intended to cause. But I was about to discover that I was holding onto something, of which I had been completely unaware.

"Where are you?" Chris asked as she directed me to travel back to where my emotions were keeping me "stuck".

"I'm standing on an icy road," I replied, the words leaving my mouth only then making me aware that I was back at the scene of my miscarriage "and I can see my car crumpled against the tree".

"And what are you feeling?"

"I'm relieved. Oh my God, I feel guilty because I'm relieved about losing my baby!" Chris gradually brought me back into the present moment as tears streamed down my cheeks.

"I had no idea," I stated, shocked at the information I had just discovered. I had always thought that the guilt I felt was due to being responsible for causing the miscarriage.

"It's okay," Chris reassured. "Your soul knew that if you hadn't lost the baby you would be walking a very different path now. The accident was supposed to happen and you don't need to feel guilty anymore".

It defied all logic that such a traumatic time in my life could have been freeing me up to allow me to find my purpose. It defied logic; however, I knew at a deeper level that it was true. And I felt grateful. Did that mean that every trauma I had experienced up to now had been breaking me down enough to breakthrough? Somehow I felt that to be the case. Believing that, would make any future difficulties so much easier to face, because I'd know they would be making me stronger too. I had no need to feel guilty anymore. Everything really did happen for a reason. I had spent most of my life fighting myself, it was time to give in and forgive myself instead – time to step out of my own way so that I could achieve whatever it was that my soul had in store for me. I smiled to myself as I remembered the poem I had written a few years earlier about my internal battle. I could finally add the last verse;

I was searching and now I am found;
I am not my possessions, body or mind.
I am a spirit, life, heart and soul,
I am integrated, connected and whole.
I am free, awakened anew,
I am ready for true living – are you?
I am eternal, happy and me; not a dichotomy,
for I can just "BE".

I finally had the strength to acknowledge what a victim I had allowed myself to be. I no longer needed to defend myself from my shadow; it was time to accept the whole of me. I had spent years desperate for someone to save me from my pain, whereas now I knew that the only person who could save me was me – *all of the old clichés were true!* If only we were taught this in childhood; how to self-love, how to live with no regrets, and that we are all capable of healing ourselves. *Is this the biggest secret known to man?* I wondered. It was high time that it was no longer a secret.

FOURTEEN

RECOGNISING SIGNS
AND REAL MAGIC

*"If you are always trying to be normal,
you will never know how extraordinary you can be."*

MAYA ANGELOU

I had an insatiable appetite for spiritual knowledge. For the first time in my life I'd devour a book within a couple of days. I needed information to corroborate my experience and I wanted to gather as much as I could. One such book, which was to act as a torch for guiding me out of my own "fogginess", was aptly called *Out of the Darkness* by author Steve Taylor. Steve, a senior lecturer in Psychology at Leeds Metropolitan University, had collated accounts of people who had also experienced a spiritual awakening. It documented their journeys through the darkness, and out the other side, and so many of the stories resonated deeply with my own experience. Somewhere I had read the phrase; "When the pupil is ready, the teacher will appear" and Steve's appearance in my life at that time through his words on the page, felt like a wish-granting genie appearing in a puff of smoke from a magic lamp! *This is what I want to be able to do for people by telling my own story one day,* I thought. I messaged Steve at the email address at the back of the book and thanked him for writing something which helped me to "normalise" my own experience. I no longer felt so alone, and that was vital in helping me keep myself on the right side of the sanity fence.

Since my awakening there have been amazing synchronicities happening in my life regarding people, with whom I have come into contact. At a soul level I know that these encounters are not just pure chance. It is all part of a bigger Universal plan beyond my control. Some things I can't yet explain, but I feel that "knowing" is enough, and don't always need an explanation anymore. Despite that, I have spent the last two years researching spiritual experience and dipping my toe in the reactionary water by speaking more openly about my new beliefs. Some attempts at putting my message across have been successful and welcomed, others have not; that is all part of my journey and learning to understand that not everybody will be ready to hear something that could potentially threaten their own sense of stability is all part of it. When I meet people who "get it", I cling onto them for dear life – it feels like clinging on to an oxygen mask when submerged in a sea of disbelief and misunderstanding.

One key "oxygen person" was my new friend Linda. She had just gone through a very similar experience in her own life when we first met. Ironically I had gone to her for what I thought was relationship counselling, but it turned out that the Universe had other plans for our connection. Having such a profound spiritual awakening experience which completely changes the way you see the world can be a very lonely place to be, and when you come across someone who understands a very strong bond is instantly created. These bonds hold a deep understanding beyond the brain or the conventional norm. They defy logic and can drive you to distraction if you attempt to make sense of them; most people unfortunately discover that the hard way within our current narrow-minded social conceptual frameworks, and end up in the mental health system. Linda and I instinctively knew that we needed to develop a network of peer support, people with whom we could meet regularly and share the kind of experiences that you couldn't normally share without being looked at strangely or considered to be completely bonkers. I persuaded Linda to set up a group in her cosy little counselling space, which she willingly did, and intuitively called it "Unleash my Spirit". Attending Unleash every Tuesday evening after work, (where I now felt unable to be my true self), was like having a little sanctuary for my soul amidst the insanity of the outside world. A core group of fellow "experiencers" had developed, drawn together synchronistically by profound shared experiences, and although our journeys had been very different from each other, we had now reached the same conclusion; nothing in life was certain and anything was possible. Being in that room was the most comfortable I had ever been in my own skin. I looked down at my hands and exclaimed;

"I'm in my body!"

In that moment I realised what it actually meant to be

disassociated; my body and soul had literally been disassociated up until that point. It was another light bulb moment. Nobody looked at me strangely or questioned what on earth I meant; there was just an air of acceptance for whatever was going on for me in that moment.

One Tuesday evening as I drove around the corner to park up and head to group, I was drawn to a woman walking away from me down the road. I did a double take as if I recognised her. Nope, never seen her before, I must have been mistaken. However, the minute I poked my head into the room to beam "Hello!" at my fellow "Unleashers", I spotted the mysterious woman sitting there. How bizarre I thought, it was as if I had recognised her before we'd even met.

A few weeks later we were discussing the *Celestine Prophecy* by James Redfield. It was a well-known spiritual book written as a story but documenting stages of the awakening process written as a series of "insights" taken from an ancient manuscript found in Peru. I had heard of it a few years previously, but it hadn't meant anything to me back then. Now it all made perfect sense. The first insight was having a sense of "restlessness", a kind of underlying "knowing" that there is more to life; I could certainly relate to that having initiated my journey! Then, it said, comes the awareness of more and more coincidences, chance encounters that seem to hold a deeper meaning – check! The Third insight documented a heightened perception of the beauty of nature, and the ability to see energy fields around plants. *That happened to me the other day!* I remembered. I also remembered thinking my eyes must have been playing tricks with me at the time. I could relate to each insight, pretty much in the order they were documented, and it was reassuring to hear my fellow group members say the same. We may have all been at different stages of our journeys, but the mutual support was always equal.

Linda had the experiential guidebook, a sequel to the *Celestine Prophecy* series, and during one Unleash meeting had decided it would be good to try out a few of the exercises in it for fun. We partnered up and I sat opposite the woman whom I thought I had recognised a few months earlier. The lights were turned down and we were instructed to go into a meditative state, but instead of closing our eyes as usual, to focus intently on the eyes of our partner. As I stared straight ahead the outline of her body completely dissipated into the room and all that was left were two bright lights where her face once reflected back at me. I sensed an energy come close to me, as if it was crouching at my feet and almost felt a pressure leaning on my lap.

She needs to know I'm proud of her. Tell her she's doing well and tell her to remember making rum balls at Christmas by the open fire, and mention a mole on my left earlobe. It's all going to be okay, all is well.

When our awareness had been gradually brought back into the here and now in room I recounted the information exactly as it had come to me. It had clearly been this woman's mother, who had died years previously, coming through to pass on her reassurance. Shivers went down my spine; this wasn't something I could choose to ignore anymore, I really was getting messages from spirit. Not only had I had confirmation that the message I had somehow "picked up" was very real, I now also realised that I had indeed recognised this lady – not from this lifetime, but from a previous life. She was a soul group connection. *How was I able to understand things that made no sense to my logical brain?*

Another lovely lady from our Unleash group, Suzanne, had been raving about a friend of hers who practised chirology, Johnny Fincham – a modern day palm reader. I was intrigued and made an appointment to see him. *Was there something in the way the cells in our bodies evolve over time that can allow a total stranger to read what we have experienced in life, and to even predict what may be to come?* As I pulled up outside Johnny's house I felt a mixture of excitement and hesitation. Although this kind of stuff was becoming more and more my "normality" these days, I was still a bit worried. *What if he told me something I didn't want to hear?* The next hour went by with me in a state of constant exasperation. *How on earth could this man, who knew absolutely nothing about me, read such minute detail about my life from the shape of my hands, the lines they contained and the texture of the skin?* It was completely astounding. He told me the fact that my little finger was set low down compared to the rest of my fingers was symbolic of the fact that my mother figure had been emotionally absent during my childhood. Amongst other completely spot-on intricate details about my character and history, he told me that I had an alien-like perception; that I could walk down the street and sense things about people that even they might not know! It was actually a relief to hear this being acknowledged; it was something I had known but tried to ignore. It made life difficult sometimes, especially with partners when I had tried to tell them things they weren't ready to hear. *I really did need to learn to keep my mouth shut!* Johnny told me that I was going to write a book, that it would have a "zany narrative" and make quite an impact. *How on earth did he know I had been thinking about doing this?* Now I knew I needed to stop thinking about it and get on and do it! When looking closely at the tip of one of my fingers through a magnifying glass Johnny suddenly exclaimed, "My goodness you've got a radial loop, that's quite rare! I've only ever heard of Doris Stokes and David Blaine having them before". *Doris Stokes?* Blimey! Those familiar shivers were back.

With my regular meditation practice, came increasing connection with the spiritual realm. It was quite addictive as I was receiving more and more clarity that I was on the right path in believing in my sixth sense, but I knew that I needed to be careful not to overdo it, I knew only too well that there was a "dark side" to all of this, even though so far I had been lucky enough to evade it. One young man who attended our Unleash group was always recounting experiences with dark spirits, and seemed plagued by their presence in his everyday life. He too had fallen foul of the mental health system, and he was clearly petrified of ending back up within it. He viewed Linda as some kind of saviour; she had been the one person who had enabled him to speak openly about his spiritual experiences without judging or pathologising him, and, as the months passed, his confidence to express himself in the group gradually grew. He spoke about "needing the outlet", and was clearly benefitting, as we all were, from the mutual, non-judgemental support which allowed us to integrate our "unusual experiences" into our everyday lives.

One evening I got my first little taster of an experience with spirit that wasn't quite so welcome. I no longer watched much TV. I found it on the whole depressing and I had chosen to only focus on positive things now as I completely believed that was the best way to keep my own vibration (spiritual energy) as high as it could be. Every time the news came on, relaying more bad news of some kind or other, I made a conscious effort to switch off. However, I had been unable to avoid the fact that a young girl had gone missing and there was a massive hunt going on for her. Because I didn't want to know the gory details, I hadn't turned the TV on for days. Instead I focused on *Positive News,* a newspaper, to which Linda had introduced me, thinking how much better I felt, both emotionally and physically, by making a conscious effort to surround myself with only positive people and experiences.

Sitting on my meditation beanbag that evening, I lit a candle as usual and stared into the flame. *Thank you for my wonderful journey*, I said to the Universe in my head before closing my eyes and taking three deep cleansing breaths. My head was clear of thought, something which now came fairly easily to me, and no sooner was there space in it a name was "dropped in". A name and two words: "blackened heath". As soon as I opened my eyes I realised what this message related to. I had tried to ignore it but it hadn't worked. If spirit wanted me to have a message then I was going to get it. *Maybe it was just my brain playing tricks with me – maybe it was my Ego wanting to solve a crime and there wasn't really anything in the words I'd got?* I hoped that was the case. The alternative petrified me. These weren't the kinds of messages I wanted to receive. I wanted nice flowery messages from loved ones who had passed, wanting to pass on reassuring messages to those they had left behind. But choosing what I received wasn't an option. The name meant nothing to me. *Maybe if I searched online and came up with nothing I could forget about it and put it down to my head playing tricks?* I decided to do that. I typed the first name and surname into Google. And there it was – a person clearly named in the search party of this missing child. *Shit. Now what was I supposed to do? Call the police and tell them I'd had a message from spirit telling me a name I thought may be involved in the disappearance of the missing child that was all over the news?* They'd think I was completely insane and probably arrest me. *But what if I did nothing, and later found out that this named person had somehow been implicated, and I'd done nothing about it? Shit, shit, shit.* I had no idea what to do for the best. So I slept on it and confided in Linda, I knew she was one person who would believe me and give me sound advice. Between us we decided the best thing to do was to anonymously email the police headquarters that was dealing with the investigation. I knew that keeping what could be such vital information to myself could be fatal. So I emailed the station and passed on the information. Again I held my breath as I pressed "send". I hoped that the response would be as open-minded as the one I had received from Professor Chris Cook.

A couple of days later I had already forgotten about the email. It was done and things were happening at such a fast pace my brain couldn't keep up with assimilating all of the information. Linda had invited me to attend another group being run by a friend of hers, Dawn Chrystal. Dawn identified as a medium and she talked a bit about her own background.

Dawn explained that she had always been spiritual, that she had been able to "sense" things from an early age. This evening, coincidentally for me, she focused on recounting an experience she'd had years previously with a "walk-in-angel". Dawn explained that she had been in a very bad place emotionally at the time, and had asked on numerous occasions for a way out of her life. Dawn then told the group the whole story.

Driving along one night on her own her vision became

blurred, as if she was looking down a tunnel of water. That was all she remembered as the next thing she'd woken up in the car, having crashed into the barriers at the side of the road. The ambulance driver had apparently told her how lucky she was to be alive. She recounted feeling blessed in that moment; feeling that the accident had come along to shake her out of her depressed state. However, for weeks following the accident, Dawn went into what she described as a "comatose state". She said, despite feeling emotionally fine in herself now, physically she felt drained of energy and was virtually unable to move, although there hadn't been anything evidently wrong with her. The hospital had put it down to shock, but she explained that as time went on, her symptoms did not improve, that she felt somehow detached, as if she were looking out from the chair in which she was sitting through someone else's eyes. She said that she felt as though she didn't belong in her own house, and she looked around as if her surroundings, (where she had lived for years), were unfamiliar, somehow. After a couple of months of being pretty incapacitated Dawn realised that there must be something deeper going on. She recounted asking spirit to help her in finding out what was wrong with her, and it was then that she was able to find a way to release herself from the situation. She told us that she discovered that her body had been taken over, at the time of the accident, by another soul; a "walk-in-angel", by the name of Mary. Mary had been disabled when she was alive, and bound to a wheelchair.

I shivered as I listened to Dawn continue.

Dawn said that Mary hadn't wanted to leave the earth plain, and that when she'd heard Dawn's wish for a "way out", she'd seen it as an opportunity for a "way in". Dawn had subsequently visited a spiritual healer and been assisted to communicate with Mary, asking her to leave her body. Mary had apologized and Dawn now saw it as one of her many learning experiences; that we should always be mindful of what we wish for, because the Universe is always listening in one way or another.

The point of Dawn recounting her story that evening had been to demonstrate how important it was to protect ourselves from spirits, which was apparently even more important if we were emotionally vulnerable or an "empath" (very sensitive).

As Dawn spoke I was mesmerized. *Maybe it was possible that Mum had been taken over in some way, as she had always felt, by a spirit during the time of her second suicide attempt. That would explain an awful lot. She wouldn't have known about protecting herself, and she had been emotionally very vulnerable at the time.*

When I returned home that evening I had received a reply from the police in response to my email. They had taken me seriously and passed on the information to the investigation team. Again I breathed a huge sigh of relief. *It was time for me to start taking all of this more seriously.*

I'd had another kind of vision and this time it made me chuckle. Not the kind of vision where I actually hallucinated, (although I could see it happening in my head), again it was more of a kind of "knowing" and difficult to put into words. I had been thinking about how this spiritual stuff desperately needed to be normalised and spoken about openly, both on mainstream TV and radio. *Where better would it reach most people who were probably in need of it being acknowledged than on breakfast telly?* The thing that made me chuckle was the fact that I saw myself sitting on the couch with Phillip and Holly having a general chat about my experiences like it was the most natural thing in the world. The weird thing was I actually knew it was going to happen! Again, I confided in Linda – I knew she wouldn't laugh at me, well not about that anyway. I said to her, "All jokes aside, how many people must be suffering in silence without access to information or a peer support group of like-minded people like we have?" This really was life and death stuff. I knew that there were a few clients I worked with who were feeling suicidal, I suspected, for similar reasons. We were so very lucky to have "found" each other. I suddenly remembered what Mum had said to me that day I had raced to see her from Wales when she had got readmitted to hospital; "I saw you on the telly"... What if she had been experiencing some kind of premonition? I now knew that there were lots of documented reports about the existence of pre-cognition; that it was actually possible to know something before it happened. I really did need to do more investigation around this.

I had been in regular communication with the Spiritual Crisis Network (SCN) since my first contact with them after speaking to Marie and finding out about the founder, Catherine Lucas (author of *In case of Spiritual Emergency*), the previous March. Because of this I had now been invited to their AGM. I felt honoured, but slightly apprehensive. I asked Linda if she was interested in attending it with me seeing as she'd also experienced a spiritual crisis, so we both headed down to Brighton to meet the team. The meeting was being held in the home of one of the development group members, a wonderfully welcoming lady, who herself had experienced a spiritual crisis, as (we later discovered) had the majority of the team. The meeting was chaired by Isabel Clarke, and I discovered, to my disappointment, that Catherine Lucas was no longer actively involved. I had been hoping to meet her and share my wonderfully synchronistic story of how I had been introduced to SCN by our mutual friend Marie. *If I hadn't been brave that day and confided in Marie about my experience, I wouldn't be here,* I mused. I was in awe of Isabel. She was a Clinical Psychologist based in a London NHS Trust but was pushing conventional boundaries with her determination and apparent passion to make the mental health system more open-minded when it came to "anomalous experiences". She talked about "shared reality" and "unshared reality" and it was like music to my ears. Linda and I agreed to take part in the training to become volunteers to answer email requests that came in to the network; requests for support, like I had made the

133

previous year, from people who were struggling to understand and assimilate their spiritual experiences. It was the least I could do in the circumstances – SCN had played such a vital role in enabling me to understand and cope with my awakening, and I wanted to be able to offer the same support to others in need.

During the training Isabel talked about how it was vital to be able to keep "a foot in both worlds" of shared and unshared reality, and that it became dangerous if a person were to stray too far into the "unshared realm" as this is where they can become completely disassociated and lost "beyond the threshold". This made perfect sense to me as I had intuitively known that meditating too much could push me over the edge of insanity, so to speak, and I made a mental note to stay as grounded as possible within shared reality. The training was straight-forward enough, and contained sound advice. I was impressed at how such an unusual subject could be dealt with so "matter-of-factly".

It turned out that Isabel hadn't actually experienced a personal spiritual crisis like the majority of the other development group members, but had instead come to work in the mental health field later in her career, after studying the history of mystics and prophets. Due to her in-depth knowledge of this, she had been able to equate the "mad ramblings" of her psychotic clients to the experiences often described by prophets in historical literature, and had come to her own, unconventional, conclusions about what was actually going on. Her tenacity and willingness to stand up and defend the underdog only made me admire her even more. I wanted to be part of the SCN family, I felt like I had come home to the fold and I'd do all I could to help spread their invaluable message.

After the training I could be officially added to the development group list, where I would get to see email requests for support coming in from not just the UK it turned out, but all over the world. It felt amazing and I was very proud to now be on the road to offering support to others who were also experiencing something similar to what both my mum, and myself, had experienced. It felt surreal, both in a fantastic and immensely scary way. Life was, I was beginning to realise, one great big bloody paradoxical experience.

Synchronicities were now a part of daily life. I'd get signs that I was on the right path in one way or another, either through words that spoke to me at a profoundly deep level, even if they were displayed on a run-of-the-mill notice board, or through numbers that had a certain significance. It's difficult to articulate exactly what I mean unless you have experienced something similar, but the best way to describe it is that "magical" occurrence when something happens that makes your energy soar in a completely natural way, without any need for external influences. I have since heard it referred to as "being in the flow", and this is a perfect way to describe the feeling. One such example was when a friend happened to mention the books by Brian Weiss. The first one I read was *Many lives, many masters*, where Dr Weiss talks about his experience as a Psychiatrist performing regression therapy on his patient, Catherine, who actually started to recount numerous past lives. In his books he talks about how he has discovered through performing his own regression therapy, about reincarnation and past life soul recognition, and as soon as I read this I instantly knew that that had been my experience that day with the lady from my *Unleash* group. It had been inexplicable at the time, but now I had an explanation. We had known each other in a previous lifetime, and had met again as we still had lessons to learn from each other. This stuff was truly magical, and as I received clarity, my vibration soared.

I now know that the Universe speaks to me, in various ways. I watch out for synchronicities and follow my instinct and intuition as I know full well that it leads me down the right road, even if my logical brain tries to fight it sometimes! The Western brain has not been raised to understand telepathic experiences, energy or pain exchanges, or soul recognition. At least not yet. I am hoping that this will change within my lifetime. One step at a time is the only way – and I know patience is one of the lessons. There are lots of lessons to be learned on a spiritual journey, but once you become consciously able to manage them they can actually become quite fun! I soon discovered that the more I looked for answers the less I found, so I realised that I needed to let go of searching and let the information find me when the time was right – the Universe has a plan and it was going to put that plan into action in its own time frame, not mine! Although I know that, my Ego often complains and gets impatient – it wants to control and continues to search. Only now it doesn't take me long to realise that all this achieves is to prolong the time it takes for information to come my way!

So, now I knew my experiences were absolutely and undoubtedly real, but I also knew that if I was to convince the "unbelievers" I needed hard evidence. Hard evidence in the form of science. *Urgh.* Science had never been my strong point. But now there *was* a point, like never before, to gather as much information as I could – and that is exactly what I intended to do.

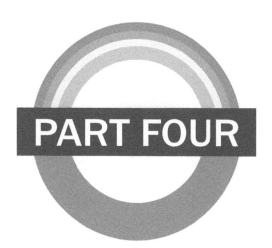

PART FOUR

BREAKING
THROUGH

COLLECTING EVIDENCE AND MAKING A DIFFERENCE

"Whether you think you can,
or you think you can't, you're right."

HENRY FORD

For a year or so I had been incessantly trying to get my foot in the door of my local NHS Trust. Having built up a pretty good working reputation with my colleagues in the locality, I was in a lucky position to attempt to get the statutory services to listen to the need to acknowledge spirituality within their work. Interestingly, I discovered there had actually been quite a few previous attempts in Norwich. After numerous emails to an influential person within the Trust, regarding the new spirituality strategy they were developing, in which I told him that I was a member of the UK *Spiritual Crisis Network* and could be of use to their strategy development, I managed to wangle myself a meeting. I knew how important it could be to so many patients if I could convince them to take spiritual crisis seriously (it was after all a category in the *The Diagnostic and Statistical Manual of Mental Disorders (DSMIV)* – "Religious and spiritual problems") and now I had a chance to be heard. Talking about Mum's and my spirit experiences was clearly way beyond his comfort zone, but I was now able to be compassionate to this, despite my desperation to get my point across. When it was suggested that there was no way anomalous or paranormal experiences could be acknowledged within the strategy guidelines as it was just too "way out", I knew I had only one chance to get my point across;

"Let me try to explain the distress caused when you experience a spiritual awakening, an expansion of consciousness, and nobody believes you. It's like knowing that you're gay but not being able to live as a gay person. Having a spiritual awakening and not being able to openly live a spiritual life would be the same as a gay person being forced to live a straight life, it's just impossible. It becomes intrinsic to who you are."

I could see that I had touched on an emotive subject. I had been heard. It would take time to build up trust and prove that I was grounded enough to be of assistance, but that was okay, I had made a start and that was enough for now. I was actually proud of myself. *What a strange feeling,* I thought as I walked away, tears of relief welling up in my eyes. Never before would I have dared to even speak to a person of such importance, I would have felt too insignificant and inferior. My old, "I can't do it", limiting beliefs had been replaced by thoughts of "I can do it!"– this negative to positive thought-changing malarkey really did bring about better outcomes. I had made a conscious effort to put into practice what I had learned on the Mindspan workshop, in addition to repeating daily positive affirmations as Louise Hay's books suggested and, even though I had felt like a proper plonker doing it, the benefits were now starting to show. It really was possible to change your own neural pathways – I needed to look more into how this worked. Now I believed I had something to offer, I had knowledge that could help patients who were suffering in the same way my mum had, feeling unheard and possibly being misdiagnosed and over-medicated due to being misunderstood by a system that was yet to evolve itself, spiritually. It was going to happen, and I would be part of ensuring it did. Suddenly the message I had channelled about being a vehicle to relay a message (to change the conceptual framework around mental illness) didn't seem quite so unachievable. I had started to build a bridge to *Mend the Gap.*

I had also built up quite a rapport with the hospital chaplain, Ted, since my initial contact with the Trust – I knew SCN would be easily forgotten if I didn't keep pestering them to acknowledge the vital work we did. The staff needed to know about it as a resource and somehow I'd find a way to get it mentioned within the spirituality strategy practice guidelines. Ted was writing the guidelines and I liaised with him to ensure SCN got a mention. I'd developed quite a soft spot for this chaplain. He had a glint in his eye and, despite not really saying much about his own beliefs, I just knew he "got it". I found it absolutely bizarre that I felt a kinship with a man who represented religion. I had always recoiled from anything to do with religion previously, and it frustrated me that people seemed to equate being spiritual with being religious. To me religion was just the cause of war, and it made perfect sense that the only reason religions exist was because they had evolved within different cultures attempting to make sense of, and put their own conceptual framework around, the spiritual experience. To me religion was the complete opposite of spirituality – it served only to separate people into fundamentalist and reductionist factions, whereas spirituality, despite being a very subjective experience, was all-encompassing and expansive. I think that's what I loved about Ted; he never preached, and his mere presence was soothing in some way.

I had been attending the Trust's spirituality strategy public consultation meetings as a way of keeping my own presence felt. Eventually it had been recognised that, despite my beliefs, I was actually fairly sane and seemed to know what I was talking about, and so I was invited to speak a little about the work of the *Spiritual Crisis Network*. Now I really felt as though I was getting somewhere. That evening I made an excited phone call to my parents. I had been keeping them regularly updated on what I was doing and hoping to achieve and, although not totally understanding the scale of the difference I was hoping to make, it was clearly having a positive impact on their own self-belief and our relationship. Since my own epiphany I had been openly discussing my spiritual journey and insights with both Mum and Dad, and encouraging mum to be more open about her own journey. She really struggled to have the confidence to speak about her own experiences, not surprising after having spent so many years having to keep it all quiet. I knew that I had to prove to her that it would help her to talk, and that she needed to be able to integrate her truth with everyday life. It was a momentous task for someone who had been forced to deny herself for so long, and she was clearly petrified that if she began to talk more openly she would be considered to be becoming ill again. Not only did she need to express her truth, but she also needed to start releasing deeply repressed emotions that had been stunted for literally the whole of my life due to her medication. She had a huge journey to make, but with my new insights into how to support her differently, I was able to journey alongside her and reassure my dad that it was okay to just let her "sit with" any emotions that arose. And they did. Huge waves of emotion that took us all on a scary rollercoaster ride. Despite the challenge of managing this without medical intervention, we were all becoming closer. I was less defensive and better able to express and manage my own emotions, and so I was better placed to be a support to my parents, to whom this was a completely new world of "being". Our relationship was blossoming; Dad was getting his wife back after years of living with an emotional robot, and underneath it all we knew that what was to come was worth the years of hidden pain. It was all going to be okay; all would be well.

The other character, for whom I had developed a real soft spot, was Isabel Clarke, one of the SCN directors. Her feisty nature would have, at one point in time, terrified me, but now I could see that driving it was her soft heart and a rampant desire, equal to mine, to get spiritual crisis openly acknowledged and appropriately supported within the mental health system. I respected Isabel's intellect and endless knowledge in addition to her tenacious spirit and so was honoured when she invited me to run a workshop at the Spiritual Crisis Network conference in Sunderland that June, to be entitled "Finding Solid Ground". My hard work and persistence to get SCN firmly on the map was paying off. I had taken SCN's own advice and stopped meditating so regularly – continuing with yoga and weekly group meditation sessions seemed to be the right mix for me to maintain my own internal balance.

As I planned the slides for my presentation, the magnitude of how far I had come since feeling so lost and suicidal only four years previously hit me. I was sensitive, but now that I knew it was good to be able to express my emotions, I shed more tears of happiness and gratitude, which was actually much healthier than keeping them bottled up. I allowed my happy tears to freely flow.

My presentation was entitled;

Taking Spiritual Crisis into the NHS at the front door.
How professionals and experiencers can get the NHS to acknowledge the importance of including spirituality in their work
With the footnote;
Katie Mottram: Worker within the Mental Health Services, Experiencer of Spiritual Crisis.

I was "outing" myself publicly for the first time, and it was a real test as to whether my bravery could outweigh my fears.

One of the keynote speakers at the Finding Solid Ground conference was Dr Charlie Heriot-Maitland, a Clinical Psychologist at Kings College London, and colleague of the Spiritual Crisis Network, whom I was very proud to know. Charlie initiated his presentation on the outcomes of his research study entitled *Helpful versus unhelpful psychotic experiences* with the question "What do you think makes the difference between exceptional / out-of-the-ordinary experiences (OOE) being manageable and beneficial in ordinary life, and being unmanageable and leading into mental health services?"

Charlie had interviewed two groups of people, a non-clinical group (NC), meaning people who described having OOE's but had avoided coming into contact with mental health services (like me), and a clinical group, meaning people whose experiences had been pathologised and treated as an illness (like my mum). His conclusions exactly matched the experiences of Mum and me:

Summary of findings
- Group similarities
  - Triggered in context of negative emotion, often accompanied by isolation and contemplation about meaning / direction of life
  - OOEs provided emotional fulfilment, and insights

revealed were meaningful in the context of emotional concerns (fulfilled a psychological purpose)
- Breakdown of conceptual ego boundaries → new conceptual outlook
• Group differences
  - NC group had more prior conceptual knowledge, open attitudes, and receiving validation and acceptance from others
  - NC > C perceived desirability and transiency
  - C less appraisal options and more urgency

Charlie went on to discuss the implications of his findings;
• The contextual factors triggering an OOE are different to the contextual factors involved with incorporating an OOE
• An OOE itself is not pathological; to the contrary, it is adaptive and generally enhancing
• The "pathology" is when the purpose and meaning of the OOE is failed to be acknowledged through lack of integration with inter-personal and background personal contexts
• Bio-psycho-social models need refinement; i.e. OOE vulnerabilities separated from clinical vulnerabilities
• Associating OOEs with clinical psychosis may be detrimental
• 'Radical normalisation" and emotional validation in clinical work is needed.

Yes! It all made perfect sense! Finally this stuff was getting the recognition it warranted within a statutory setting. With research evidence like this, spiritual experiences could no longer be ignored in psychiatry as being too "out-there". Changes were beginning to happen and I was excited to have a front-row seat.

I was now starting to become more interested in the body/mind connection as I couldn't help but notice how much better my own health had been since my emotions were more stable. Everything was synchronising; body, mind and spirit. Knowing how important it was to have, not only precious relaxation time in order to give my poor little brain a well-earned rest, but also time alone to enable me to listen to my soul in order to keep me on track, I booked myself a week in Crete. It was also a kind of gift to myself, time to assimilate my new knowledge and to prove that my confidence had now developed enough to allow me to go on holiday alone and actually enjoy my own company. I had planned to do absolutely nothing but swim, sunbathe and enjoy some "down-time". Nobody really knew quite how much work I'd been doing in addition to my conventional full-time job, and keeping my spiritual life pretty much separate from that was taking its toll. This was a week where I could be completely true to myself, there was no need to hide anything as nobody would know me.

Settling down into my seat on the plane I plugged-in my earphones. I had bought the audio book, *The molecules of emotion* by Candace Pert and, after watching the clouds disappear below the plane wings, I closed my eyes to listen. I thought this might dissuade anyone from talking to me as I didn't really feel like making small-talk with a stranger just to be polite. Candace was talking about opiate receptors affecting the bio-chemistry of the brain and the limbic system, (which was connected to the threshold of the emotions of pleasure and pain), in relation to consciousness, and I suddenly realised that being spiked with Angel Dust might have initiated a shift in my inability to manage my emotional thresholds (leading to my suicide attempt) and began the expansion of my own consciousness, which was then heightened by activating my pineal gland when I started meditating. I needed to find out more about the science behind spiritual experience – it was fascinating! The refreshment trolley clattering along the aisle woke me from my musings and I turned to the gentleman sitting next to me. I'd better make an effort to make conversation if I expected him to pass over my drinks order. We exchanged a few generalities about how nice it was to get away from the British summer weather and where we were staying. Then he asked me what I was planning to do with my week.

"Oh, not much," I replied, "just lots of reading, swimming, lying in the sun, probably a bit of meditation." I hesitated at the last admission; I wasn't usually so open about my spiritual practice. I hadn't realised how much being ridiculed for it had affected my willingness to be so honest. *I need to get over that, sod what anyone else thinks, I know the benefits!* I thought to myself. "Oh you meditate do you?"

prodded my new friend. *Here we go, more ridicule.* "My wife's just getting into that", he replied, and as if on cue she leant forwards and nodded enthusiastically. Okay, it was safe to carry on talking. "Yes, quite a lot actually, and practice yoga, I'm really interested in spiritual development".

"It sounds as though you two need to sit together" he laughed, as he motioned to his wife to swap seats with him. For the next two and a half hours Patricia and I exchanged stories and she confided in me that she had always known, since childhood, that there was more to life than she was being told, that Western society was missing something meaningful in some way, and it had left her feeling a bit lost, incomplete somehow, and grappling with depression. I told her about my dreams to get the mental health system to acknowledge spirituality, and to write a book about my experience, in order to normalise the spiritual experience in Western society.

"Oh you have to do it!" she exclaimed, "I'm so pleased we met! You've inspired me to believe in what I'm doing, and I'm going to order the books you've recommended as soon as I get home."

What Patricia didn't realise was that her honesty in telling me how much my own story had given her hope, gave me the confidence I needed to continue with my own dreams to speak openly about my truth. It was proof that it worked and was needed. *Thank you, Universe, for another synchronistic meeting and mutual life lesson opportunity*, I said inwardly, as the plane touched down and the welcome sun warmed the side of my face through the window. *Let there be light!*

And there was light during that week, in all kinds of forms! The sun shone brilliantly every day and my intuition was on fire – I was most certainly "in the flow"! I was relaxed, and able to be in the moment every minute of every day, focusing on my breath, the sand between my toes, and the salt on my skin as it dried after swimming in the sea. I had taken another book to read, *Stepping into the Magic* by Gill Edwards – and it was such a fitting and pleasurable read. Gill had also taken a leap of faith to write, which increased my confidence to follow my spiritual path, and I decided that week that I would, when the time was right, leave my job and focus on what I knew my soul yearned to do. It was a scary prospect, but the excitement and natural energy that the decision created within me overtook my fears. I hadn't intended on doing any work that week, but planning a workshop flowed so effortlessly that it didn't feel like work at all. *If I could do this and make a living then I never had to feel like I was working ever again. Gill was right, it felt like pure bliss!* I'd create the slides for my workshop when I returned home, but that would be easy now all of the planning had been done. It was all coming together; I had managed to synchronise myself, and so I'd call my workshops "Synchronise You!"

My determination to research the science behind the connection between the body, mind and spirit was now even stronger. I had to find evidence for the existence of consciousness beyond the brain and the effects of our thoughts on our biology, not only to get the doctors in the Trust to take me seriously, but also because that would be what my workshops would focus on. I checked my emails and there was a circulated advert from the SCN development group about the British Congress on Medicine and Spirituality, to be held in London in October. *I had to go.*

Ted, the Trust chaplain, had introduced me to one of the Psychiatrists who had spoken to him due to a particular interest in spirituality. Yasir and I met to discuss our mutual interest and what had led us to our beliefs. Yasir was involved with the Trust's spirituality strategy development; as he had suggested that it was intrinsic to psychiatric care, and because of his own passion, he arranged a debate to discuss how integrating spirituality into clinical work could improve service quality and service user experience. I was honoured to be invited as a representative of SCN to argue in favour of spirituality being included in care-planning. Following the debate there was a write-up from Yasir in the Trust magazine;

Hellesdon debates are new learning experiences that we would like to incorporate into the regular weekly postgraduate teaching programme for doctors in Hellesdon Hospital. These sessions will aim to explore controversial topics in psychiatry and stimulate thinking about different principles and practices. I chose the first session to be on spirituality due to the recent drafting of the Trust's first strategy on spirituality and also due to the importance of this topic when providing care in culturally diverse settings.

Due to the success of the debate, Yasir asked if I would be interested in providing a presentation to the doctors as part of their extra-curricular training, based on the science of spirituality. "It wouldn't be until early next year though," he said. *Perfect I thought, just enough time to collate the evidence I collect from the British Congress.* And inside I did a little excited dance. "Absolutely", I replied. "It would be my pleasure."

My excitement reached fever pitch as I travelled down to London on the train a month later. However, despite being overwhelmed with just how quickly my spiritual journey was travelling, I was able to contain my excitement with a paradoxical sense of calm. *It was all fine; everything was happening just as it was supposed to.* I took some deep breaths and repeated to myself; *All is well.* This time I was attempting to get my head into the right frame of mind by reading Bruce H. Lipton, PhD's *The Biology of Belief* (www.brucelipton.com). I had come across his amazing work about epigenetics via a YouTube link on Facebook, the only place where I was overt about my spiritual beliefs and so did most of my networking with like-minded people all over the world. I wasn't interested in most of the banal gossip that went on over the site, but for literal Universal connection it had been invaluable. I thought about how much I hated technology when I first had my awakening. I had wanted nothing to do with materialism of any kind, craving a simple life with nothing but nature. It hadn't been easy, but I had managed to integrate my new-found beliefs back into modern day life as much as possible, and I could now see that technology was actually part of the evolutionary process. Everything is constantly evolving, and science was now catching up and beginning to prove some of the things people had known, but been unable to prove, for centuries. My thoughts turned back to my book. Bruce was talking about the emerging science of epigenetics. He was postulating that epigenetics was one step "above and beyond" genetics, and this emerging science was disproving that we have to be controlled by our genes. Bruce had discovered, through years of research that was pushing the boundaries of conventional science, that our thoughts really do affect our physiology because of the different brain chemistry that is released into the blood depending on whether our thoughts and consequential emotions are either negative or positive. I had read quite a few accounts of self-healing, and now the science was proving how it worked. Miracles are real life! I thought, as my energy soared once more. Thinking about how old mysteries were now starting to be proven reminded me of when I had first come across the spiritual teacher Louise Hay before my own awakening experience. She was famous for having channelled the information for her book *Heal your mind, heal your body* from spirit decades ago, and was now a worldwide, well-respected figure in the spiritual teaching circles. *Wow*, I thought, *how amazing to think she knew stuff all those years ago that nobody believed. How brave of her to have spoken out about it.* I wondered whether the world would be so evolved now if it wasn't for people daring to be so outspoken. I knew Martin Luther King was right, but I also knew the thought of actually doing it was petrifying.

Sorting out the reams of notes I had taken at the British Congress, I wondered how on earth I was ever going to sort them into any kind of comprehensible presentation. I flicked through, circling certain key points with different coloured pens to try to indicate to myself how relevant they were and how they interconnected. When I was at school I never for a million years thought that I'd be doing something like this by choice. Words like "psycho-neuro-immuno-endocrinology" would have been complete gobbledygook to me a few years ago, but now I wanted to tear the words apart and examine their entrails. I wanted to understand; I intuitively knew stuff, but my brain needed to catch up. I was now equipped with the evidence I needed to prepare my first official solo presentation: "The science of spirituality; creating a new paradigm". Because of my own experience, and through the research I had done, I knew that it was possible for absolutely anybody to experience a spiritual awakening, that nobody is immune, and so being equipped with prior knowledge was the best form of preventing the experience from turning into a crisis – but would the doctors be ready to hear this? How ironic it was to think I'd be openly saying, to a room full of around thirty psychiatrists, the kinds of things my mum had said to one doctor which had led to her being sectioned all those years ago. *But this time I'd be armed with evidence and so I'd be safe... I hoped so anyway. Now really was the time to pray!*

As I stood at the front of the projector in my suit and heels, (although I didn't believe it was important what I wore, it was a well-known fact that people made a judgement of you based on appearance within the first few seconds), my legs felt like jelly. *This is for you, Mum,* I thought, to take my mind away from what seemed like hundreds of pairs of eyes staring straight at me. I felt like a lamb, offering myself up for slaughter. I smiled and introduced myself to the room. I told the doctors that only five years previously I had been actively suicidal, had no confidence and felt unworthy of living. I told them that this breakdown had led to a "breakthrough" for me, in the form of a spiritual awakening, and that I had taught myself how to turn my life around without any need for hospitalisation or medication. The next hour passed in a blur as I relayed the information from my *PowerPoint* slides. I told them that the term "spiritual crisis" / "spiritual emergency" was coined by Stanislav Grof and his wife in 1989, and they defined it as *Critical and experientially difficult stages of a profound psychological transformation that involves ones entire being,* and that Carl Jung had first referred to a breakdown as potentially leading to a "breakthrough". I told them that in the early 1990s authors Lukoff and Turner made a proposal for a new diagnostic category entitled "Religious or Spiritual Problems", and that the category was approved by the DSM-IV (the psychiatric diagnostic bible) Task Force in 1993. They had cited that:

- Non-ordinary experiences and psychological disturbances can overlap
- Western medicine may have different and potentially conflicting values about patient experiences.
- People need specialised support when in spiritual crisis.

I told them that I was a member of the UK Spiritual Crisis Network development group and that we provided this specialised peer support via email to anybody who wrote in.

I looked up; nobody was looking horrified or holding up a straightjacket, so I continued.

Next was my slide entitled *An evolutionary shift.* I told them that I believed, as Dr Larry Dossey, (a Texan Pharmacist and author of *Reinventing Medicine*), had said, that we were moving into a new age of medicine. Dr Dossey had coined the term "non-localised mind", meaning that the mind exists beyond the brain, and stated in his book; *I used to believe that we must choose between science on the one hand, and spirituality on the other, in how we lead our lives. Now I consider this a false choice. We can recover the sense of sacredness, not just in science, but in perhaps every area of life.*

Dr Peter Fenwick, (Neuropsychologist, Lecturer and Consultant at Kings Institute of Psychiatry), had been a keynote speaker at the Congress, and he had a particular interest in research into near death experiences. This research was starting to provide evidence as to the existence of consciousness beyond the brain. During his talk Dr Fenwick had said something that resonated deeply with me. He'd said that we need to bridge the evolutionary gap, that there is no longer "animate" and "inanimate" matter as we now know that everything is energy. Ignorance of this in the modern era is what creates huge fear. He believed that a re-conceptualisation of consciousness beyond death would reduce this fear. A new conceptual framework – *I was standing here in front of a room full of doctors who were listening to me speak seriously about the words I had channelled from spirit. Woo hoo!* I looked up again; there was nothing like a reminder of how much fear I felt in that moment to regain my composure. Dr Fenwick's suggestion was that existential questioning is the basis of all distress due to the fear of death. It made perfect sense to me – it was this existential questioning that I had done since childhood that had caused my own depression. Now I knew that the mind and the brain are not the same thing; that there was research to prove the existence of consciousness beyond the brain, and it meant that I was no longer scared of dying. I was just energy in human body form; my soul was eternal. I told the doctors that other doctors, like them, had also written about their own experiences of this phenomenon –

Dr Brian Weiss, the American psychiatrist who had been made aware of past-life recollection through a patient of his, and another American, Dr Eben Alexander, who had written about his own near death experience whilst being struck down with a near-fatal bout of rare meningitis. I reminded the doctors that we could all learn from each other, and that learning through shared life experiences was sometimes more valuable than conventional education. *That might have been pushing the bravery a little too far!* But I was on a roll...

I recounted other evidence that I had gathered for the existence of consciousness after clinical brain death. Dr Penny Sartori, once a Welsh-based intensive care nurse, had conducted a five year clinical study on the near-death experiences of her patients. She had concluded that when in cardiac arrest, the brain function deteriorates within eleven to seventeen seconds, due to blood flow interruption, but patients had been revived and recalled experiences despite being classed as brain-dead well beyond that time frame. The only scientific and logical explanation for this was the existence of consciousness outside of the brain – the "non-localised mind". I also told the doctors about AWARE, an international study initiated in 2008 by Dr Sam Parnia of the Horizon Research Foundation, who qualified at Guys & St Thomas hospital, now the Director of Resuscitation Research and Assistant Professor at the State University of New York. Author of *The Lazarus Effect; the science that is erasing the boundaries between life and death.* The AWARE study includes pictures being placed on shelves over resuscitation beds, only visible from above. Early reports taken from resuscitated patients detailing what the pictures depicted suggest that the mind operates in the absence of brain function.

I noticed some of the doctors shifting uncomfortably in their seats out of the corner of my eye. Looking up again I smiled to reassure them that it was nothing to be afraid of. *How could this be happening? It was so surreal!*

I threw in the names of another few eminent doctors who mooted the same theory. Dr Giancarlo Lucchetti from Portugal had been a speaker at the Congress and had said, "The brain is merely a tool for the manifestation of the mind". Dr Carlos Roberto de Oliveira, (an anaesthesiologist), corroborated this, describing the brain as a kind of "radio receiver" that picks up consciousness and translates it according to individual human experience: "The mind is not a product of the brain – it doesn't produce but transmits information." As I read this out it reminded me that during my epiphany my brain had been awash with infinite information – Universal consciousness. In some way my brain had been able, for that short period of time, to stop filtering and just allow everything in. *Surely this had to be what psychosis was about – the brain being overloaded with information that it doesn't have the capacity to logically process.*

"So," I asked the doctors, "could mental "illnesses" actually be manifestations of something beyond the brain, and not brain dysfunction? Now I was getting into the realms of psycho-neuro-immuno-endocrinology. Could the pharmaceutical industry be defunct? Except I didn't say that last bit; I thought that would definitely be a step too far, for now anyway.

Dr Roberto de Oliveira had talked at the congress about a Brazilian study into trance states (meditative practice), that indicated less brain activity via an MRI scan when a person was in trance state, but they had heightened cognition. This was proof enough that their cognition was coming, not from their brain, but from beyond their brain.

Dr Mario Beauregard, a Neuroscientist and Researcher at the University of Montreal, had also presented his discoveries in the neuroscience of emotion at the British Congress;

"There is now much evidence to counteract the reductionist theories that there is no correlation between the body and mind (thoughts/emotions)..." he had said. *Yes! I had thought at the time, I knew all of this was true!* He had taken MRI scans of research-study subjects during meditative states and these scans demonstrated reduced activity in the amygdala and hippocampus areas of the brain, which lead to states of emotional calm and a homeostasis in the body. By purely thinking happy thoughts the subjects serotonin levels increased; Dr Beauregard had shown how the placebo effect has a positive impact on the physical body. As he talked it also confirmed why my repeated affirmations had had such a profound effect on my own brain. I had heard of neuroplasticity before, but now the theory made complete sense. The repetitive use of positive affirmations create new synaptic connections changing the structure of the brain, and improved neural pathways allow more positive instinctual responses, emotionally and physically. Positive emotions are proven to boost the immune and endocrine systems. By ignoring the fact that I felt like a plonker and doing my affirmations anyway, I had helped to heal my brain and body – *not such a plonker after all.*

I thought this would be a relevant place in the presentation to include a bit about what I had learned from Dr Candace Pert in *The molecules of emotion.* Dr Pert had discovered through outcomes of one study she conducted that there is a chain reaction of neurotransmitters from the brain that attach to "hot spots" in our body and penetrate the cells there – these "hot spots" are dependent on what emotions initiate the reaction. These findings substantiated the teachings of Louise Hay, who experienced cervical cancer in relation to her own repressed emotion following a rape. Louise had healed her cancer through healing her emotions relating to the cause. Dr Pert hypothesises in her book that the amygdala stores emotional memories and sends projections to the hypothalamus to activate the sympathetic nervous system: a fear response is initiated, heightened by negative held basic self-beliefs. Cortisol, the fear hormone, is released, and if there is prolonged exposure to this the immune system is damaged leading to a dysfunctional autonomic nervous system...This quite literally causes dis-ease in the body.

Nobody was saying anything, but as far as I could make out, nobody had gone to sleep either.

I carried on talking. My legs had stopped shaking and I had actually started to enjoy myself. The next slide explained, what I believed, to be the cause of emotional dysregulation;

- From conception, stress hormones affect a baby's development and levels are set at six months. If exposed to heightened cortisol levels when the nervous system is developing it can damage the activation and efficacy of the parasympathetic nervous system (the bit that helps us to calm down), therefore meaning memories can be stored incorrectly and "Fight/Flight" reactions are triggered more easily.

- If over-exposed to stress the developing amygdala becomes sensitive and over-active (common in highly sensitive people with traumatic backgrounds)

Could this be one causation for people who are diagnosed with unstable emotional personality disorder? I postulated. It had been my experience when working with people who had this diagnosis, that they had all experienced difficult childhoods. It would have been quite possible for me to have received this diagnosis at the time of my suicide attempt, I mused. Thank God I was lucky enough to have been living outside the UK at the time. *Where might I be now if I had been diagnosed and unable to self-heal?*

The next statement was the crux, as far as I was concerned, of my whole presentation;

- HOWEVER; ALL DETRIMENTAL PSYCHOLOGICAL AND PHYSIOLOGICAL DAMAGE CAN BE REVERSED ONCE THE PINEAL GLAND IS ACTIVATED – This is why meditation and spirituality plays such an important role in modern medicine!

In 1945 Sir Alexander Fleming sparked an interest in the pineal gland, a tiny gland at the centre of the brain. In 1948 Chico Xavier, a Brazilian Medium, controversially channelled theories about the pineal gland in relation to mental health and was subsequently accused of being mad. *Nothing has changed in over sixty years, I thought, it was about time it did.* However, he bravely wrote books about his theory of consciousness channelled from spirit and worked with open-minded scientists who made advancements beyond their time due to the information he relayed regarding melatonin having a role on cognitive function. Forty years later his theories were proven to be true.

Now I was treading on very dangerous ground; I had gone from speaking about hard science to openly talking about channelling messages from the spiritual realm, and I was in a room full of psychiatrists; *I must be absolutely bonkers!* But I'd come too far to stop now. I continued...

Some of Dr Julius Axelrod's (a Biochemist who worked at the National Institute of Mental Health), later research in the 1960s focused on the pineal gland. He and his colleagues showed that the hormone melatonin is generated from tryptophan, as is the neurotransmitter serotonin. The rates of synthesis and release of these hormones follow the body's biorhythms in harmony with the hypothalamus. Dr Axelrod and his colleagues went on to show that melatonin had wide-ranging effects throughout the central nervous system, allowing the pineal gland to function as a biological clock. The pineal gland is known as the connection between our physical bodies and the spiritual world, and is why it is common for sleep patterns, the aging process and body temperature to all be affected when the pineal gland is activated through meditation/spiritual practice or sudden awakening. I remembered how I used to wake frequently in the middle of the night around the time of my own awakening, and how my body completely changed – my nails and hair even seemed to grow at an amazingly fast pace!

I reiterated to the doctors that it is suggested by researchers of "Conscious medicine" and Epigenetics that all detrimental physiological damage can be reversed through meditation and conscious intention. I suggested they might like to watch the film *What the Bleep do we know?* which is based on the new discoveries of quantum physics, including "the observer effect" which offers proof that dematerialises our current world view. There is now scientific proof that humans are not powerless biomedical machines; we can actually be conscious creators of our own reality – all we have to do is believe it! I had not only read the science of epigenetic mechanism through the work of

Louise Hay, Candace Pert, Gill Edwards and Bruce Lipton, I had experienced my own proof – since I had healed my own repressed emotion I had not been ill once, and as soon as I developed a little sore throat or tweak of a pain in my knee I knew that it was my body trying to tell me that something in my emotional state wasn't quite right. This really was body/mind/spirit connection – intricately linked and inter-related. Quantum physics describes each and every one of us as having a bio-energetic vibration on the magnetic spectrum. The Heartmath Institute has deduced that receptor proteins capture vibrational energy fields within a twelve-foot radius, and this is how we can "sense" someone's frame of mind or the "mood" of a crowd when we walk into a room.

The work of Dr David Luke, Lecturer in Parapsychology at the University of Greenwich and also a keynote speaker at the British Congress, intrigued me. He had carried out studies on the neurochemistry of altered states of consciousness. As per the findings of Dr Mario Beauregard, the MRI scans in Dr Luke's studies had indicated reduced frontal lobe brain function during trance states, despite reported increases in experience. He gave the example of a psychographer, (someone who channels written words from spirit), writing when in a meditative state: "There is a direct correlation between anomalous experience and reduced brain activity that logic cannot comprehend."

I knew this had to be true. The information I had written in my theory during my awakening had been beyond that held by my brain. The words had flowed through my hands as if from somewhere beyond myself.

Dr Luke explained that these scan results displayed a similarity to the effects of Psilocybin and other psychedelic drugs on the brain. It seemed likely that meditative states turn off the restrictive brain "filters", opening us up to Universal consciousness when the pineal gland is activated in the same way as when ingesting drugs. A Peruvian drug, dimethyltryptamine (DMT), commonly known in South America as "the drug of the spirit: Ayahuasca", causes a polymerase chain reaction. This amplified DNA sequence was improved by Dr Kary Mullis (molecular biologist), who won the Nobel Prize in 1993 for his studies using psychotropics. *Why had this information been around for so long, but was so little spoken about?*

I concluded my presentation with various research studies, examining the relationship between psychosis and spirituality, and the detrimental effects that pathologising anomalous or "out-of-the-ordinary" experiences can have. I quoted one of my favourite phrases from one of Isabel's books, *Psychosis and Spirituality, consolidating the new paradigm*:

Science cannot replicate subjective experience; knowing the anatomy of a bat does not give us the subjective experience of what it feels like to be a bat.

The stance of SCN is to look at the validity of treatment for those who consider their psychosis to be spiritual in nature. There, I'd managed to get in another mention of SCN.

I also added the overall conclusion of Dr Charlie Heriot-Maitland's *Helpful v unhelpful psychotic experiences* research study which he'd published in *The British Journal of Clinical Psychology 2012 Vol 51, 1*, the thing that had stood out to me at the SCN conference the previous year.

Radical normalisation and emotional validation in clinical work is needed.

I told the doctors, who still seemed to be listening to me, that I was excited that Charlie had been awarded funding for a three-year research study into the clinical validity of the support offered by the UK SCN;

"I know this to be vital through my own personal experience", I found myself saying. I had found my own voice independent of my slides.

"We know through new scientific findings the validity of the placebo effect. It therefore stands to reason that there is a "Nocebo" effect; that giving a negative prognosis and dysfunctional diagnosis is detrimental to the recovery process, psychologically and consequently also physically. It really is time for a new paradigm for psychiatry".

I thought I'd better close with a few names they'd know, and no doubt respect more than anything I had to say. I told them one of my favourite quotes from Dr Andrew Powell at the 2013 British congress on medicine and spirituality;

It is the fate of the awakened mind to fall foul of societal confines as it knows no boundaries.

How could they argue with the words of such a well-respected Psychiatrist?

"We are coming out of a secular era where science has been confined to the physical Universe, which has created fear and instability. Einstein proved that time and space are merely local phenomena, but there is existence beyond local phenomena and when this veil is lifted the mind perceives what science is still, and has yet, to discover".

And I knew nobody would have the audacity to question the words on my final slide;

The measure of intelligence is the ability to change. Albert Einstein

I knew that I'd never been the most intelligent pupil in class, but I had an open-mind, and I now knew that counted for more than being arrogant enough to think that I had all of the answers. Nobody has all of the answers as new discoveries are always being made and life is in a constant flux of change. *Maybe I wasn't quite so stupid and insignificant after all.*

SIXTEEN

NOBODY IS IMMUNE!

"Listening has the quality of the wizard's alchemy.
It has the power to melt armour and to produce
beauty in the midst of hatred."

BRIAN MULDOON

Over the last couple of years I have been honoured to make connections with some truly inspirational people who have either experienced their own spiritual awakening, or are open-minded enough to want to acknowledge and educate around the importance of the phenomenon and its implications. They all know that anyone can experience a spiritual crisis, and that it is therefore much healthier to be forearmed with information.

None of us know all there is to know, that is certain, but united we can come closer to the truth. All of the following wonderful people chose to contribute a piece especially for Mend the Gap as they also have a desire to connect, collaborate and share the same vision for positive change. When we lower our egoic defences and take on information that challenges our "limiting beliefs", it allows us to truly connect and transformation occurs.

Synchronicity led me to the following individuals, who each express their unique viewpoint as to why it is so vital that spirituality is acknowledged within psychiatry.

171

I'll let the wonderful Steve Taylor PhD, (a senior lecturer in psychology at Leeds Metropolitan University, and the author of a number of books on psychology and spirituality, including *Back to Sanity* and *Out of the Darkness* – www.stevenmtaylor.com) explain the phenomenon to kick off:

There's a popular belief that the state of being "spiritually awakened" is a wholly blissful experience, a state of perfect serenity and equanimity, in which all problems and anxieties disappear. But my research suggests that this isn't usually the case. Although people who go through the process of awakening do experience enhanced well-being, and in most cases eventually reach a state of serenity, the initial stages of the process can be extremely difficult.

"Spiritual awakening" usually means the dissolution of a person's normal "self-system" or ego. Their normal sense of identity is disrupted, even broken down, and is replaced by a new "self-system", with a new identity. (In my book Out of the Darkness, I compare it to a butterfly emerging from a chrysalis.) Often, the dissolution of the normal "self-system" is brought about by intense psychological turmoil and trauma, such as bereavement, serious illness or disability, the end of a relationship, loss of a job etc. Usually when these events occur, they simply cause a breakdown, but for some people – a minority – they can bring about a

"shift up" to a higher state of being. A latent, higher-functioning self emerges, to replace the old identity which had dissolved away.

The dissolution of the old self and the sudden emergence of a new "self-system" can be very disruptive. People who go through the process are sometimes confused or even bewildered by their transformation. Strange new energies may be released inside them which cause psychological and physical difficulties. They may have difficulty sleeping, feel unexplained pain and discomfort throughout their body. Their previous, stable well-organized mental functioning may be disrupted, so that they find it difficult to function in day to day living. They may have difficulties with concentration or memory. These difficulties usually fade over time, so that eventually the new state of being usually does become stable and integrated. But in some cases, this can take several years, or even longer.

The real danger here is that these difficulties will be mis-diagnosed as psychosis – an error easily made by psychiatrists who aren't familiar with the process of spiritual awakening. If the experience is pathologised, and if the person is given medication to control their symptoms, then the natural stabilising process may be halted, so that he or she becomes "stuck" in the difficult or disruptive phase.

It's my belief that there are many thousands of people whose spiritual awakening has been mis-

diagnosed as psychosis and who are suffering as a result.

What people who undergo the process of spiritual awakening need is understanding and support. They need a framework to make sense of what is happening to them, to make them aware that they're going through a process which, no matter how difficult and disruptive it may be, will eventually lead them to a higher and deeper state of being.

This is exactly the kind of understanding and support offered by the Spiritual Crisis Network, (www.spiritualcrisisnetwork.org.uk), of which Isabel Clarke is a Director. Here she reiterates why it is so important that the journey is supported;

Spirituality can be understood in terms of a sense of relationship with that which is beyond. The individual might label this as relationship with God, Spirit etc, or by some vaguer concept, but since this concerns a way of knowing that is beyond words, names are unimportant here. All relationship belongs to this way of knowing; that is, knowing not by propositional knowledge, but by visceral experience (Clarke 2010 pp 105-6).

Furthermore, as human beings we are only partly self-contained individuals. Our apparent autonomy needs a fabric of relationships and roles to sustain it.

It is all too easy for that fabric to become disrupted. Because of the idiosyncrasies of the human mind, where the person feels under threat in the present, past threat is added to the load produced by loss or change, hence the impact of past trauma on present functioning. Where this happens, things feel unmanageable and unbearable and people cope as best they can. Some withdraw and shut down (depression); others maintain a state of ruminative hypervigilance; yet others, who have this facility (the high schizotypes), access another dimension, where infinite, usually unrealizable, possibilities, anomalous experiences and paranoid terror beckon.

This emotional and experiential overload obliterates problem solving capacity, and self-defeating coping, such as attempting suicide, resorting to alcohol or drugs etc. replaces this. At such times, the individual often needs to reach out to a widest circle of relationship to get some sense of containment and coherence – the relationship with that which is at once deepest and furthest; the spiritual/religious dimension of relationship (Clarke 2008).

Where the support provided by social context and particular helpers enables the individual to navigate this breakdown as a journey towards a fuller experience of self and of life, breakthrough to a deeper understanding, reached through stepping temporarily beyond the bounds of the self, is possible. This might be seen as a spiritual journey; a spiritual crisis. All too often, the journey is brought to a halt by undiscriminating use of medication and the person's sense of themselves is shattered by stigmatising labels.

Clarke, I. (2010) Psychosis and Spirituality: the discontinuity model. In I.Clarke, Ed. Psychosis and Spirituality: consolidating the new paradigm. (2nd Edition) Chichester: Wiley

Clarke, I. (2008) Madness, Mystery and the Survival of God. Winchester:'O'Books.

I feel so blessed to have found support not only through the *Spiritual Crisis Network*, but through Linda, a friendship which turned out to be mutually-supportive. Linda explains her experience of spiritual awakening:

As I stepped out of my favourite chair in the conservatory it was like I was stepping from a heavenly new world. I felt that I had been floating on a cotton wool cloud and wrapped in luxurious soft silk and bathed in a warm glowing light. As I actually stepped back onto the cold kitchen floor, I realised I had been in a trance-like state and now I was seeing the world, society, money, the medical system and even my long harmonious marriage, with a whole new perspective, in a totally different light. It was like I could see right into the very core of everything; like I had taken off the wrappers and could see the naked essence of truth in every person, relationship and dynamic. My values turned upside down in a moment and my heart was bursting with euphoria. I felt powerfully compelled to express and act on my new values and intense feelings, yet I could hardly believe the words coming out of my mouth. Could everyone be right? Was I being irrational, psychotic, mentally unbalanced, ill, even though I felt so alive, free and full of love?

The chaos that ensued was dramatic and culminated in me moving out. Over the next few months, I gradually felt the pain that I had caused to my family; my empathetic insights were like a series of gunshot wounds to my heart as I realised the impact of my decisions on those I loved. I felt alienated, scared, despairing and alone.

After triggering such suffering for my family, I made it my passion to find out exactly what had happened to me. My years of personal development studies supported me, but did nothing to explain my experiences. I studied psycho-spiritual counselling and Spiritual Companions at the Mangreen Trust, which validated and affirmed my experiences and provided a framework for understanding. I am hugely grateful for the sacred space for deep reflection and support from Naomi and William Duffield at Mangreen. The validation and acceptance I received, inspired my Unleash My Spirit group, so I could support others in a similar way: it is now associated with The Spiritual Crisis Network.

Spiritual awakening can rock your world, and the deep bliss and psychotic-like experiences can be followed by confusion, intense emotional outbursts, instability, paranoia and fear, especially when you realise you still have to organise practical stuff, talk to "normal" people, go to work and pay bills.

Key to integrating my experiences and making my life work in a more coherent and powerful way, has been the Mindspan programme. Although I was generally familiar with the content, Gavin Drake, has developed a system of powerful principles that are easy to digest and apply in every day situations. Its simple practicality, was the difference that made the difference.

Immersing myself in Mindspan turned out to be a gift of recovery and supported my reintegration into a focused and fulfilled life, where I am feeling more present, alive and engaged than ever. Forgiving myself for those decisions and choosing a healthy focus has empowered me to be more responsible for the consequences of my decisions and enhanced my sense of inner peace. Drawing on the thinking competencies has been like an architecture for empowerment, so that I am navigating the ever flowing rhythms of life with a sense of stability, purpose and happiness, totally assured that I am living my best life and bringing my potential to the fore.

As Mindspan has been so key to my recovery from crisis, I have made it my business to share it with others, encouraged again by Katie's success in applying the principles so diligently and whole heartedly. Experiencing her integrating her experiences and insights gradually into a focused, practical way that brings such a powerful and valuable contribution to the shift in psychiatry has been truly heart-warming and awe inspiring.

She has mastered responding to life so that she knows she need not suffer and so continually learns and grows. Her courage to consciously create and choose her life path is constantly inspiring and I feel honoured and blessed to have been her house mate, best friend and soul sister!

Linda Allen
linda@mind-span.co.uk
(www.mind-span.co.uk)

Rachel Miller, who is considered an 'Expert by experience' due to her personal experience of having her emotions labelled, demonstrates the devastating effects of being diagnosed by the current mental health framework, and how alternative belief systems can impact so much more positively to the outcome:

At the age of eighteen, I was diagnosed with bipolar disorder. During the depressions, I have not wanted to live in this world. It felt too full of hate and anger, everything that is harsh. I felt too sensitive and fragile to survive in it. However, at other times I was so moved by beauty, art, music and nature that I felt as if heaven was on earth. I felt so much energy and passion for life. But, I felt at the mercy of my emotions, like I had no control over my life. I struggled to remain employed as my emotions would overwhelm me and I was constantly anxious and having regular panic attacks.

Three years ago I became involved with a spiritual development group and since then, I have gained great understanding of these experiences. My teacher described the depression as the "Dark Night of the Soul". My true self was longing to emerge. I had been rejecting my true creative passions and sensitivity, suppressing it in order to fit into a societal role that I was expecting myself to fulfil. I desperately wanted to be like everybody else-to hold down a nine-to-five job, to have a car, a yearly holiday, enough money to have the luxuries in life. I desperately wanted love and approval. But my soul was screaming out for nature, meditation, art, music, writing, spirituality. I thought these things would make me an outcast and that I wasn't good enough. Suppressing my true self was causing a dark depression to cast over me. My soul needed me to make changes.

Through the weekly spiritual and personal development lessons I learnt that my extreme sensitivity to the emotions of others can be explained in terms of clairsentience – I energetically "pick up" the emotions of others, like a sponge or a magnet. Our teacher takes us through energetic exercises that focus on recognising which emotions belong to us and which to other people. The exercises are performed in meditation and involve grounding and centring our energy, and clearing any energy and emotions that do not belong to us. These exercises have been like magic! I always feel so much clearer and stronger after performing them, which I now do regularly.

We also identify thoughts and beliefs which are not serving us in life and learn to change these to positive ones, through meditation, journal-writing, practice and patience. We are learning to love, forgive and accept ourselves, as well as other people, just the way we are.

Spiritual development has allowed me feel in control of my life again, and no longer at the mercy of my emotions and thoughts. I have gained the courage and empowerment to change my life in ways which allow me to live as my true self and, because of this, I have so much more hope for the future.

Dr Mick Collins, now a well-respected lecturer of Occupational Health at the University of East Anglia and recent author of *The Unselfish Spirit: Human Evolution in a*

Time of Global Crisis, describes his own journey through spiritual crisis;

> *In the early 1980s I lived for just under three years in a Tibetan Buddhist monastery in the North of England. I attended the Buddhist teachings and meditated daily. At one point during my stay I decided to visit some friends in the West of England. On the train journey I was quietly reciting mantras when I had an overwhelming experience of love and compassion for all the people on the train. The experience continued and became more intense. When I got off the train I was experiencing pulsating waves of bliss throughout the whole of my body. Moreover, inanimate objects and people appeared to me as though they were sacred. The experience lasted just over two days. It was a profound spiritual encounter unlike I had ever experienced before.*
>
> *However, not long after this intense mystical experience I started to feel quite unsettled and was not prepared for what happened next. I experienced a Kundalini opening, which resulted in feeling intense heat around my navel, coldness below my knees, a low-level vibration throughout my body and a pressure around my forehead. The experience turned into a spiritual crisis and included strong feelings of anxiety and agitation. I sometimes felt as though I were caught in a conflict between good and*

evil, *often feeling consumed by violent thoughts and projections. Extreme impulses, turmoil and panic would flood into me, and I was not able to carry on with my usual routines and interests in daily life. I spent two years (unemployed) trying to work through the psycho-spiritual complexities the experience uncovered. In the next paragraph I will plot my journey through the spiritual crisis and I will link key developments to publications I have written on the subject.*

1. *Once I had worked through the aftermath of the psycho-spiritual challenges from the crisis, I had the idea of wanting to work with people. I studied for a diploma in health Science and then trained to be an occupational therapist. I worked in an NHS acute admissions mental health unit and started to integrate spirituality into my therapeutic practice.*

2. *Also, at this time I spent nine years training in transpersonal psychotherapy and eventually worked in a specialist NHS outpatient psychological therapies team. Throughout my time working as a therapist, I worked on building my skills and understanding to help people explore their human potential, listening out for opportunities for healing and growth.*

3,4. *Spiritual crises are difficult to manage and they certainly can be painful, but they are also transition points for further psycho-spiritual development.*

5,6. *I have written elsewhere about the collective potential that spiritual crises may have as tipping points for transformation.*

7,8. *That is, they may help us recognise that we are living in a global state of emergency.*

9,10. *Due to climate change, decreasing natural resources and a growing world population. Spiritual crises may well be the psyche's "sane" response to our current unsustainable ways of living in the world, which is becoming increasingly unbalanced.*

11. *Thankfully **nobody is immune** from spiritual crises, and these experiences may be most important in helping us all wake-up to the planetary crisis we are facing.*

1. *Collins, M. (2008). Spiritual emergency: transpersonal, personal, and political dimensions. Psychotherapy and Politics International, 6(1): 3-16.*

2. *Collins, M. (1998). Occupational therapy and spirituality: reflecting on quality of experience in therapeutic interventions. British Journal of Occupational Therapy, 61(6): 280-284.*

3. *Collins, M. (1999). Quantum questions: the "uncertainty principle" in psychiatric practice. Part 1. Holistic Health: The Journal of the British Holistic Medical Association, 61, 21-24.*

4. *Collins, M. (1999). Quantum questions: the "uncertainty principle" in psychiatric practice. Part 2. Holistic Health: The Journal of the British Holistic Medical Association, 62, 21-23.*

5. Collins, M., & Wells, H. (2006). *The politics of consciousness: illness or individuation? Psychotherapy and Politics International, 4(2), 131-141.*

6. Collins, M. (2007). *Spiritual emergency and occupational identity: a transpersonal perspective. British Journal of Occupational Therapy, 70(12): 504-512.*

7. Collins, M., Hughes, W., & Samuels, A. (2010). *The politics of transformation in the global crisis: How spiritual emergencies may be reflecting an enantiodromia in modern consciousness. Psychotherapy and Politics International, 8(2), 162-176.*

8. Collins, M. (2008). *Politics and the numinous: evolution, spiritual emergency, and the re-emergence of transpersonal consciousness. Psychotherapy and Politics International, 6(3), 198-211.*

9. Collins, M. (2010). *Global crisis and transformation: From spiritual emergency to spiritual intelligence. Network Review. Journal of the Scientific and Medical Network, 103, 17-20.*

10. Collins, M. (2011). *The global crisis and holistic consciousness: How assertive action could lead to the creation of an improved future. In Conscious connectivity: Creating dignity in conversation, ed M. Brenner, 214-23. Charleston, SC: Pan American.*

11. Collins, M. (2014). *The unselfish spirit: Human evolution in a time of global crisis. East Meon, Hant's: Permanent Publications.*

Next we hear from another worker within the healthcare sector, more specifically linked to psychiatry, Lisa McKenna:

I worked as a mental health social worker/AMHP/ Manager/Lead for seventeen years with Norfolk County Council and Norfolk and Suffolk Foundation Trust. I am currently taking some time out in order to recharge, refocus and reconnect with my roots.

'It is no measure of health to be well adjusted to a profoundly sick society" (J Krisnamurthi).

When I was a student social worker nearly twenty years ago on my first placement in mental health services, it soon became apparent to me that psychiatry was more concerned with pharmacological "symptom control" and maintaining somewhat dubious power dynamics, than it was ever to do with health, wellbeing and recovery.

I had been on an "observational" institutional placement in a residential care home for adults with "severe and enduring" mental health problems. I spent my days with the residents drinking tea, smoking, laughing and talking. I met many sensitive, bright, funny individuals whose lives had been blighted by illness and stigma, and also blunted by the side effects of too much medication. Their "illnesses" had roots in abuse, trauma, vulnerability and isolation.

It seemed clear to me that the causes of many of these disorders were not solely medical in origin, but were rooted in trauma and crises of the spirit which could not be treated by pharmacology or understood by the limits of accepted "reality".

I was shocked and saddened that the lives of these individuals had been basically "written off" by a society which both invalidated and tried to "ab-normalise" their experiences while robbing them of any autonomy or control. As far as I could see the system was way more sick and dysfunctional than the individuals it was tasked to care for. However, this was not the fault of the psychiatrists who were often very well meaning and compassionate but appeared to be working from an outmoded paradigm which was also in sway to the powerful agendas of the pharmaceutical companies.

From that point I was drawn to working in mental health services as I had been fired by a passion to try to find ways of nurturing the spirit – by giving back hope and fostering connection on all kinds of levels to those whose spirits had been battered by both the trauma of mental illness and the injustice and abuse of a system which had a vested interest in upholding a narrow view of "normality" and "reality".

Since I had been a teenager I had been drawn to exploring and studying the mystical, the sacred and the profane in human experience and had been engaged in exploring creative, alternative possibilities and expanded realities. I had lived outside of "normal" *society for many years so could see the confines of established "truths" more clearly than some. I felt that the increasing consumerism and greed of the world we had inherited had resulted in a destructive and short sighted form of spiritual blindness causing the more materially affluent nation states to become increasingly disconnected from nature, from each other and, of course, our very selves.*

I was aware that we were – and still are – at a point of potential spiritual evolution if we choose. I felt – and still feel – very strongly that we can work towards creating a more humane and enlightened world and want to be part of the "solution" rather than contributing to the "problem". I am still, to date, working on it! We need to ensure we use our energy towards finding the best way forwards rather than criticising what came before. As Socrates wisely suggested;

'The secret of change is to focus all your energy not on fighting the old but on building the new".

Julie Leonovs, has an MSc in Psychological Research Methods and describes herself as a Mental Health User, Worker and Activist. She explains why the bio-medical model is so outdated;

Psychiatry with the medical model has placed too much emphasis on "disease", "disorders", biology, chemistry and reductionism. These factors still heavily dominate the discipline and I would argue that as a result, psychiatry and much of the mental health system has lost its way in what it means to care for the whole person...human beings. We are not just chemical and biological entities that can be separated into parts but are whole beings that at a higher level experience intense emotions, conflict and at times existential crisis. The phenomenological aspects of a person's life, their thoughts, emotions, experiences and spirituality play just as crucial a role in creating individual uniqueness. To view people as detached Cartesian beings will ultimately affect how they perceive themselves, how carers view them, the kind of help they will receive and their healing outcomes.

Crucially, it needs to be recognised that when a person experiences a crisis or long-term mental distress, this does not always amount to an internal biological fault, a "disorder" or disease of the brain – that can be sorted with a "chemical cosh". Very often a crisis has been reached due to extreme environmental antecedents and/or trauma whereby an individual becomes acutely aware of their position in the world and their widening feelings of incongruence. At times of emotional distress a person can become so isolated from their surroundings and everything they have relied on to support them (both negative and positive) that often, the only thing they *have left to cling on too is an emerging sense of spirituality and hope. If mental health workers fail to address and explore a person's trauma by explaining this away by some reductionist "internal biological abnormality" and also fail to recognise a person's spiritual beliefs, then they could potentially alienate this individual further by taking away the only hope they have left. Rather than mental health workers being fearful of a person's emerging spirituality, this should be embraced and looked upon as part of the healing journey, not some psychotic episode or an accumulation of an already diagnosed mental "disorder".*

"For a seed to achieve its greatest expression, it must come completely undone. Its insides come out and everything changes. To someone who doesn't understand growth, it would look like complete destruction" (Cynthia Occelli).

As internal conflict is safely worked through and resolutions are reached, the individual should begin to emerge with a greater sense of inner strength, understanding and peace of mind. Although life's difficulties will continue to arise, the individual should be better placed to manage such situations knowing at the same time that their faith and spirituality walks with them on their journey, not a "magic bullet" contained in a pill box or some label of a "mental disorder" given.

It is not just people in the UK who are waking up to the problems that the current mental health framework contains. I have had the pleasure of coming into contact with people all over the world through doing this work, and the Netherlands seem to be leading the way in many respects. Here Wendy Van Mieghem, Dutch Psychotherapist, writer and teacher in inner growth (www.wendyvanmeighem.com) sums up the spiritual journey so eloquently, in how it unites us all:

Life's vast tapestry of possibilities

Life is a wondrous, breath taking event. It encapsulates many polarities, as it is cruel and caring, dark and light, earthly and spiritual, creative and destructive.

*Life is a chain of present moments with an unlimited amount of possibilities. It grants us humans a full **freedom of choice** to live our lives the way we choose. Yet, there appear to be certain reoccurring patterns in the challenges we face on a universal and individual level.*

*Most people (un)consciously feel that it is not possible to open ourselves every second to the full range of possibilities life is offering us. For example, to take all risks of what could happen into account, or to leave all options open to the directions we can possibly choose in our daily lives every second. It is too stressful and demanding for our nerve system. We need to build some **behavioural, emotional and***

191

rational patterns *that we can rely on. To live life without any patterns would probably drive us mad...*

Sane or not?

So, we all tend to deny parts of our **nature of being** *to* **reduce** *the overwhelming reality as it is. We tend to structure our reality, shape it and filter it in a way that we (un)consciously choose. From this, our patterns in dealing with our instincts, emotions, feelings, thoughts and inspiration arise. These patterns are partly copied from our parents, teachers, peers, neighbours and friends.*

Whether we do or do not **trust ourselves** *in our ability to deal with emotions and with life itself, is therefore passed on from* **one generation to the next***. We mix it with a purely individual, intrinsic element that encapsulates our passion or motivation to live.*

Yet every time we **deny** *an aspect of our inner self, we become a tiny little bit* **less sane***. Every time we* **allow** *an aspect of our inner self to be present, and learn to deal with the emotions, feelings and thoughts that arise from it step by step, we* **heal** *a little bit from the inside out. We then become a tiny little bit "***more sane***".*

Throughout each day, we "normally" tend to **move in and out** *of denial of aspects of ourselves. We may also move in and out of allowing aspects of ourselves. To put it roughly: if at the end of the day or night we've allowed more than we've denied, we* **heal** *bit by bit* *through time. When we deny more than we allow to be present, we slowly become less sane. We may not notice this at once. On average it takes years before the sum up starts to affect our day-to-day wellbeing.*

Self-development *is the ongoing process of giving yourself the* **attention and time** *you need in order to heal bit by bit. It is an individual matter; no one else can do it for you. By giving yourself the time and attention you need to recover from stress and inner conflicts, you help yourself to become more aware of* **who you are** *and* **what it is that you need** *to find fulfilment through your daily life.*

Technically speaking, self-development leads to an increased awareness of our **individual insanity** *and to learn to deal with the consequences. To fully* **integrate** *the emotions, tensions and pain that is involved in healing means to learn to allow them to be in the present moment; to learn not to deny their existence. As a side effect, it brings us insights and wisdom about who we are and about life itself.*

Healing through consciousness

Reality contains many layers, as **mindfulness** *teachers are aware of. There is an incredible healing power in letting things "be" as there are, in respecting reality as it is, on every level. Reality is anchored in time and space in the present moment.*

The healing ability of the present moment is often

referred to as *"**the power of now**"*. To learn to recognize, allow and accept reality as it is, requires quite a lot of consciousness.

Practising meditation and mindfulness, preferably with the help of an experienced teacher or therapist to learn to move through blind spots as well, can help to develop and deepen your consciousness and mindfulness skills.

Not to alter or manipulate reality in any way, is often the hardest thing to do, for it demands from us to take responsibility for our emotions and patterns that are also part of the present reality.

Even though it may take years of practice to learn to deal with emotions and pain on a deeper and deeper level, the reward is as grounded as it is sweet. We learn that our instinctive reaction to intense emotions and pain is to let go of contact with that part of reality. It makes us lose contact with ourselves.

As we learn to trust that we are able to find our way through emotions without altering them, we feel more **connected** with ourselves, with others and with life itself. It helps us to find our way to **our inner home**: a safe, warm and bright inner feeling that makes us feel truly safe and at home with ourselves. An anchor that keeps us centred and balanced as we express ourselves through our qualities and are of service to others.

Trauma and psychiatry

Every intense life event, every trauma, settles in our system by the way we do or do not allow emotions, feelings, memories and underlying existential fears and doubts that are involved with this life event to be present in our day-to-day life.

The way we deal with our instincts, emotions, feelings and thoughts on a daily base shapes us. This is what our attitude towards life stems from.

Many psychiatric disorders are in my opinion in their core a mixture of two human aspects:

- *An inability, up to a certain degree, to deal with one's instincts, emotions, feelings, thoughts and inspiration in a constructive, comfortable way up to an existential level.*
- *A lack of inner trust to deal with one's instincts, emotions, feelings, thoughts and inspiration in a constructive, comfortable way up to an existential level.*

These two aspects interact with each other. As a result, psychiatric symptoms may become less or more severe over time.

In my private practice I've had the opportunity to support clients through individual psychotherapy sessions. I've seen people with psychiatric diagnoses overcoming their limitations through time, "freeing" themselves by allowing pain, emotions and patterns to be present.

195

The insights and inner wisdom that flew through them as a result, gave their self-confidence a boost. The way they experienced their daily lives altered. It became more bright and light. Through time an irreversible healing from the inside out appeared to have taken place, as if the penny dropped permanently.

But I have also seen people without psychiatric diagnoses become less sane over time, despite all efforts and best intentions. Some were just not ready yet to let it sink in, trying to postpone their inner homework. Others were having such a hard time, being harassed by inner conflicts and fears, that it fed their inner distrust. (This is why it is so vital that extreme emotion be "normalised", so that it is allowed to flow).

Mental health care systems

Clients often do not only have to deal with their own distrust, but also with the distrust of others.

All around the world there are mental health care systems that tend to deal with psychiatry by not making contact and denying one's feelings and inner truth. Every time I hear about this, I feel extremely sorry. It is painful to hear, for I personally feel making contact is, together with trust, the most healing aspect there is.

Still, in much of health care education students are taught not to make contact with their clients: they are *not allowed to show compassion or to feel touched when they meet a client. As a result, professionals are not truly able to listen to what the client experiences nor are they able to encourage and support clients to find their own way through the misty fields of inner emotional struggles.*

Professionals have learned to take over their clients' responsibility to heal. As you may imagine, taking over responsibility is a devastating act of mistrust. It expresses the (in)direct message that the client is incapable of dealing with one's own emotions, which is exactly the fear and inner doubt the client has been struggling with before they reached out for help.

As I see it, it is impossible to truly heal in this way. For a lot of the suppression that takes place by mental health care professionals comes forth out of their own inability and lack of inner trust to deal with one's own instincts, emotions, feelings and thoughts in a constructive, comfortable way up to an existential level.

Making a resolute distinction between the professional and the client, not allowing a sense of connectedness or contact, and not truly listening to what the other is experiencing and believing, is therefore "illusional" by itself.

From where I stand, there is no distinction between professionals and clients. We are all human, and we all struggle with our humanity. The degree in which we are able to deal with instincts, emotions, feelings, thoughts and inspiration varies over time and has much more to do with experiencing than with knowledge.

A true "professional" knows their limitations and one's humanity through experiences and by heart; "knowing" from the inside that there comes a lot more to true healing than the professional self is capable of. It involves life itself.

A professional can make contact, can listen and walk along for a longer or shorter while, but they can never say, "I know how to make you better" or "I know what it is that you need." (The only answer to that is within the individual themselves).

Healing is an inside job

One's healing journey is foremost an inside job. It demands one's attention, time and fine-tuning to heal. It demands someone's devotion and willingness to get to know oneself and learn to deal with one's emotions, instincts, feelings, thoughts and inspiration step by step.

It demands to get to know our individual purpose of life, in order to find inner peace. It often demands a change of attitude towards life and towards suffering, and a willingness to surrender to the present moment, here and now. It demands a certain degree of willingness to surrender to life as it is.

In my opinion there IS no distinction between

psychiatric and "normal" people. We are all human.
We all carry a certain degree of sanity and insanity
within us. We all do struggle with dealing with
instincts, emotions, feelings, thoughts and inspiration
on every level, again and again, as it tends to deepen
itself.

My final contributors both focus on how we in Western
culture can learn from other cultures' frameworks of
understanding mental "illness" and consequential care. I am
truly honoured to have their input, and believe we can learn
so much from what their research has found. Dr Natalie
Tobert, author of *Spiritual Psychiatries*, July 2014, explains
how her research into psychiatric practice in India has
proven that we must be more open-minded to alternative
conceptual frameworks if we are to achieve the outcomes we
desire within Western psychiatry;

> *We tend to assume western frameworks of knowledge*
> *about mental health are ubiquitous and fit all cultures.*
> *We export our knowledge globally, and our Exam*
> *Boards test other countries according to western*
> *concepts of philosophy and psychology. Our personal*
> *beliefs about human existence and the nature of reality*
> *are usually so strong, that it may be difficult for us to*
> *accept other peoples" beliefs as veridical.*
>
> *The new imperative within psychiatry is to*
> *acknowledge there are many ways of understanding*

the world. There is a problem within the original system of psychiatry, which seems to be culture bound and constrained within old style western thinking about the body and the self. However, interviews with psychiatrists, psychologists and doctors, presented in the book Spiritual Psychiatries suggests there are more spiritual ways of interpreting the human condition. They emphasise that people have different cultural frameworks of knowledge for understanding the human self, its faculties, and its experiences. Perhaps the paradigm shift in psychiatry is being led by practitioners from the East?

In the UK, from a multicultural perspective, new migrants tend to be judged by the dominant beliefs of the host population. This leads to problems, particularly in the field of mental health, when interpreting symptoms or prescribing treatments. New migrant populations aside, many people feel the experiences they have, and their symptoms of distress, are only understood and interpreted according to the old Western frameworks of knowledge. Things must change. The data in the Spiritual Psychiatries book supports medical practitioners and educators, towards a more holistic view of psychiatry. The principles of spiritual mental health from India are transferable, and can be used in both local multicultural and global public health situations.

There are many meanings of the term spirituality,

which include compassion, mindfulness, meditation practice, and wisdom. However, although these are excellent practices, they do not go far enough. To fully engage with the new paradigm, we acknowledge there are quite different ways of understanding the world, different ways of interpreting symptoms, and different strategies for appropriate treatment.

In future, I would like to see the practice of ongoing "cultural humility" where frontline medical and health care staff continue to ask: "what do you think caused your condition"? Medical and health care educational authorities might consider embedding this alongside training for clinical care, as well as post registration training in cultural models of health.

Emma Bragdon, PhD is the Founder/Director of *Integrative Mental Health for You*, (www.IMHU.org), an online learning centre for optimizing mental health. She is also the author of seven books and producer of films bridging spirituality and health and describing Spiritism in Brazil. (www.EmmaBragdon.com) She describes how being so much more open-minded about spiritual experiences and working collaboratively produces far more positive outcomes in South America;

Three Vital Roles Spirituality Can Play in Mental Health: From the writings of sages from all cultures we learn that the human being is made of 3 elements: physical, mental and spiritual. *Mainstream psychiatry has addressed the physical and mental but has not yet addressed the spiritual in mental health. Unfortunately, religion was given the task to address the spiritual but most religions do not show us "how to" develop spiritually—instead they give commandments or suggest supplication through prayer.*

Now, neuroscientists confirm we are wired for spiritual experiences and can achieve profound peace and joy; so it is time we enliven this innate capacity in mental healthcare through using effective spiritual practices passed down from the cultures who have developed the most effective ones.

Following are three roles spirituality plays in improving mental health;

1. *Optimizes Health*
   When we study the wisdom of the perennial philosophies, especially their historical roots in India, we learn that there are specific spiritual exercises that can help each of us attain the vast intelligence, bliss, and compassion characteristic of Self-realization.

2. *Guides One to Meaning and Purpose*
   Individuals most likely to be out of balance, mentally or emotionally disturbed, and/or lost are those who have not developed a sense of meaning or purpose in life. Helping individuals of all ages

define what is deeply meaningful and aligning one's actions with one's unique purpose in life provides ballast as well as direction and a goal. These are the wellsprings of true satisfaction in life.

3. *Provides Uplifting Contact with Spirit*
The dominant religions of the West abound in stories that depict humans communing with angels, and higher forces of intelligence, we call "God," or wrestling with the devil. Most psychiatrists are quick to invalidate or pathologise those who report experiences like hearing the voice of God. Thus, psychiatrists typically reinforce the notion that the world of spirits does not exist and those who experience communication with forces invisible to the human eye are "out of touch with reality".

Where spirituality is fully recognized within psychiatry individuals can learn how to disengage from negative social and spiritual influences and engage fully with positive influences. Since 1930, Spiritist Psychiatric Hospitals in Brazil have developed such practices to help disturbed individuals within hospitals, clinics and community centres. These Spiritists are also equipped to teach naturally gifted "sensitives" how to harness psychic abilities in service to their own spiritual growth as well as to help others. With Spiritist treatments obsessive thoughts and self-destructive behaviours are replaced by *inspiration, positivity, compassion, and skillful action.*

It may feel like mending the gap between spiritual experience and mental distress is too onerous a task within Western psychiatry, but if others have already done it, then surely we can learn from them? All it means is being brave enough to let down our defences and believe that another way, a way that challenges our current concepts, could actually achieve better outcomes – because they do.

SEVENTEEN

BEING BRAVE LEADS TO MANIFESTING DREAMS

*Everything your soul desires you
to be is on the other side of fear.*

The requests for support through the *Spiritual Crisis Network* were coming through regularly, from people all over the world who had realised that their mental crises were spiritual in nature, (in other words, the dissolution of their Ego), but felt alone and unheard, and had subsequently discovered the existence of the network online – I certainly knew how that felt, and it now felt amazing to be able to offer those people the support that had been offered to me when I had needed it most. I was now an official responder to those emails and regularly liaising with the development group, especially Isabel who seemed to be increasingly impressed with how I had managed to get my local NHS Trust to acknowledge the value of the support that SCN offered. They had apparently been trying for the last decade to get SCN recognised within statutory services. Isabel, who was also the chair of the psychosis and complex mental health faculty of the *British Psychological Society*, had written a couple of books about mental health and spirituality and was a well-respected speaker and author in the field. One day an email came through from her informing the group that she had been asked to write a chapter, entitled; "Psychosis as a narrative of transformation" for the next publication by the *Royal College of Psychiatrists, Spiritual Narratives in Psychiatric Practice* and asking if any of the development group would like to contribute. My heart raced with excitement and a twinge of fear that this was the opportunity for me to finally speak out publically about the experiences of Mum and I. It was an opportunity to officially be part of changing the way spirituality was viewed within mental health services. I quickly emailed Isabel back before I could give my, still very prevalent doubting-self, a chance to convince me not to do it. *This is the opportunity, for which I've wished so long,* I thought to myself, *why am I so scared?* I needed a sign that I was doing the right thing; *come on Universe, let me know if it's my time,* I said inwardly. The next morning when I turned on my laptop I saw that Isabel had replied. She told me that she was pleased that I had agreed to contribute my personal narrative. She also told me the name of the chief editor; Professor Chris Cook. I beamed and felt my energy rising again; I was back in the flow – *thank you Universe, this was so meant to be!*

I chose to believe in my soul experience, as scary as it was to do so, and the Universe was rewarding me by fulfilling my dream. Had somebody told me this would be the outcome as I sat on my bed after meditating two years previously, I'd have thought they were completely delusional – you see; life really is paradoxical. There continued to be a dichotomy happening in my life at that time. I was still working within the confines of a system where it was excruciatingly difficult not to openly discuss my experience and consequential beliefs. Now that I had settled into my own new conceptual framework for managing my life it was virtually impossible to separate that from my working environment. Each day I felt more and more as though I had to leave my soul, my very essence, outside the door of the office. I knew that I needed to be patient, and that somewhere along the line my hard work and determination would pay off, but patience for me was a real challenge at the best of times! However, now knowing that there were lessons to be learned from every difficult life situation, at some level I believed that I needed to be in my job for a reason, and that belief made staying there easier to manage. I should have known better than to question anything, let go of the need to control, and just believed that it would become apparent why I needed to be there when the time was right.

And so it did.

One of the clients I was working with at the time, Paul, confided in me during a walk one day. He told me that he had grown up with a mum who had been actively suicidal during his childhood. He was sensitive and had no confidence, and I instantly recognised myself in him. I openly told him that I had experienced literally the same thing, and although I couldn't know exactly how he felt, I was able to empathise with his situation. Fifteen years had passed since my initial worries about sharing personal information and now I couldn't care less about policy and procedure; if I knew it was going to help my client through sharing personal information then I'd damn well do it and answer questions about my professional conduct later if it arose. Experience had shown me over the years that it could be the difference between life and death. Paul and I developed a close connection over the next few months because I had given him my trust, and so he now trusted me. My instinct had been right sitting on the floor besides my young female patient all those years ago; I wished I had been braver back then... It amazed me how grateful Paul was, I hadn't really done anything, just offered him a non-judgemental ear. But it seemed to do the trick and gradually he exposed more and more of his innermost fears and emotions. One day Paul told me that he had just read a book by Eckhart Tolle. Whispering, he made sure nobody was in ear-shot;

"You see I can sense people's energies, I knew straight away when I met you that you were safe to talk to."

No sooner had the words passed his lips Paul panicked. "Oh God you're going to think I'm mad saying this." I assured Paul that I didn't think he was going mad at all, but that it would be a good idea not to tell anyone about what he was experiencing at the moment. I knew that if my colleagues heard some of these things he was telling me, he could well be at risk of having to go through a mental health act assessment, with possible dire consequences. Instantly, I found myself talking to Paul about the advice that I was now used to giving through the *Spiritual Crisis Network* about how to sit with his emotions and allow his feelings to flow, keeping himself as grounded as possible; not being fearful of his experiences or trying to interpret them too much, and learning how to discern between what his Ego was telling him and what thoughts and feelings were "heart-felt". Paul just seemed to "get it", and he and I knew that he was in the process of "waking up". I reassured him that he was going through a natural process, and that although it wasn't openly spoken about, that there were a lot of people who had also gone through it, and come out the other side. I encouraged Paul to do more reading around the subject, rather than listen to me, and to try to write a diary account of his own transformative journey, so that he could see his progress. He had been feeling suicidal, but was slowly learning not to react to these negative thoughts; to recognise that was all a part of his Ego death, and he was able to become more of a "silent witness" rather than participate in any destruction his old, basic self, was trying to cause.

Nearing the end of the project on which I was working with Paul, I felt honoured that he entrusted me with a copy of his diary, containing admissions he'd never allowed anyone else to see before. He needed to accept himself as he was, and to do this he needed to know that I accepted him, as he had been brave enough to show himself to me; completely raw. I respected his bravery so much. A few paragraphs from his writing stood out to me, (and he has given me permission to include them here, as he knows how vital it is that this message is relayed to help others like us) in his own words;

I suppose looking back I could say I had a rather traumatic childhood. I used to blame myself back then, thinking it was something I had done wrong, later to realise it was just mum's illness. I was brought up, which I can now see is like most of us, in a conditioned way. But from a young age I believed that something, somehow, wasn't right, that there was more to life. It seems most of us weren't brought up (in the West) with an open view of life, but more with one religion or another. I believe that it would lead to a much more peaceful world if children were encouraged or allowed to be more open-minded to (the possibilities of) life... Having suffered depression and anxiety for several years now and having to finish....work, it was then that I began searching for something that I had felt was always there, but at the same time not knowing exactly what.

And later on Paul described what it was like to be going through a spiritual crisis;

I was starting to see things in a new light, which I believe was meant to be as I believe everything happens for a reason. All around me my senses had become awakened; smelling, tasting, seeing and hearing – all senses in a new light. Also on meditating I was having wonderful visions, but there are some down-sides, like walking in the night (due to not being able to sleep) and feeling all the pain and suffering in the world, worrying that I might stand on and harm a living creature or cutting back plants and feeling their pain. All of these experiences my first thought was that I must be going insane, and that if I told anybody I would probably be sectioned just like my mother was. My first thought was that I had to keep quiet.... Reading "A New Earth" by Eckhart Tolle and by being open with Katie, whom I trusted, I realised that I couldn't have been further from the truth. Remember we are the sane ones, those who are choosing destruction and suffering are those in whom the Ego is in control; they are the dysfunctional ones, and it is learned dysfunction. My hope is that we will all awaken in time to save this planet from destruction. I believe there is no such thing as Heaven and Hell...we create our own Heaven or Hell within us. There's a lot about this life that I don't understand, and things are not always as they seem. I believe mental illness is part of a process we have chosen to go through in order to awaken and I believe this process can be disturbed by people being put on strong antidepressants and antipsychotics. I think the mental health experts need more education and study in this field.

There had most definitely been a reason for me being in that job at that particular time – the Universe had orchestrated mine and Paul's meeting. Now the mutual lessons had been learned, it was time for me to take my leap of faith and go it alone. I had already planned my *Synchronise You!* workshop and I wanted to put it into practice. Paul had recognised that Heaven and Hell exist within us, and I knew from my own experiences that this was very much the case. It was possible to create our own internal experience of Heaven, and I wanted to show people how I had achieved it for myself. Since my awakening, I had realised that spiritual growth and emotional growth are intrinsically linked. Focusing on personal development is not selfish, as I had previously thought, it is necessary for the evolution, not only of ourselves, but for society as a whole.

It was a few days before the launch of *Synchronise You!* , and I was going through the *PowerPoint* presentation I had planned a few months earlier looking for appropriate pictures to demonstrate the points I wanted to make. As usual, I was distracted by *Facebook*, but even that part of my life was becoming more and more integrated with work – I had made more connections online with like-minded people across the globe than I could have ever wished for pre-technological age; *I must be more synchronised now,* I thought, *I hated anything to do with technology not so long ago. How things change!* I was following more "positive daily thoughts" pages than ever, (which was another momentous change from when I used to wallow in how bad things were with the world), and one in particular caught my eye. It was a picture of Calvin and Hobbes walking along under the phrase; "I'll look after me for you, if you look after you for me."

Perfect! That was EXACTLY the point I was trying to make with the whole workshop; that by making time and effort to improve ourselves we are in fact helping each other, because if we are as emotionally stable as we can possibly be, then we don't impact negatively on those around us – which is the very thing most people are trying to avoid. *Another paradox of life. We are all so concerned with what everybody else thinks of us, we don't look after ourselves enough. Imagine if nobody in society impacted negatively on another, what a blissful life it would be...*

I continued to review the slides I had prepared, hoping that they'd make sense to my participants. I'd decided to use the analogy of a boat to explain the three parts of us – our three "selves" that we were attempting to synchronise (get working in harmony with each other). I broke it down as follows:

The Basic Self – represents the subconscious/manifests in the BODY, depicted as an anchor attached to the ship.
- Our "Basic Self" is our Inner Child and can be related to our unconscious/automatic/learnt beliefs.
- The beliefs that your basic self holds may come from your past, or even held from previous lives, and may not serve you – they can be "Limiting beliefs"

- Your Basic Self does not understand time, and experiences emotions related to those experiences as if it was "now" – this is why we get stuck in held trauma from the past and emotions can get "triggered" which in turn trigger physical reactions.
- Our Basic Self represents our physical body and the senses.
- The Basic Self reacts as if to "protect" us from new experiences – it feels safer with what is familiar, even if what is familiar does not benefit our progress – and acts as an "Anchor", keeping us stuck in the same place.
- The negative beliefs held by our Basic Self can be re-programmed and new, more positive beliefs held in their place. The Basic Self needs repetition in order to change the neural pathways, and to get rid of subconscious triggers.

I shortened the Basic Self to the acronym "BS", and thought *how appropriate, the basic self is often made up of loads of "BS"!*

The next slide explained the CS;

The Conscious Self – representative of the MIND, depicted as the main body of the boat.

- Our Conscious Self can be related to EGO – it responds to the held beliefs of the Basic self and seeks to substantiate them.
- What we believe (our thoughts) become our reality (our experiences) and this is because the Conscious Self is

controlled by the Basic self, in addition to what information it receives externally, from parents, peers, society etc.

- It acts as a "middle manager" between the Basic Self and our Higher self – which can often cause confusion and distress.
- The Conscious Self thinks, plans and is "logical". It can over-analyse.
- The Conscious Self is restricted by the Basic Self and cannot change its direction until the Basic Self changes its limiting beliefs – this is the key to releasing the anchor!

The Higher Self – representative of our spirit/soul, depicted by a sail on the boat.

- The Higher Self could also be described as our spirit or soul.
- It is the intuitive part of us, our essence, that "knows" what is best for us and our progress.
- It is the part of us that speaks to us when there are no other distractions.
- When we quieten the distractions around us we can access not only our own intuition, but Universal consciousness through our Higher Self.
- When you are "in tune" with your Higher Self and on the right path you feel energized – Your Basic Self "feels" it, even if it doesn't "know" it! – "Gut Instinct"
- Make sure you listen to your feelings– they tell you more truth than your thoughts!

- Get rid of what you "should" be thinking, and dare to follow your instincts.

The next slide depicted the three parts of us as a whole – with the anchor lifted and the boat setting sail into the distance. I found another picture to use at this point;

"A ship in port is safe, but that's not what ships are built for."

I suddenly remembered the phrase that had "dropped into my head" that I hadn't understood a few years earlier; "You can't set sail with your anchor still attached" – *Yes! It was true*; it had been a message from spirit trying to tell me that I needed to get rid of my limiting beliefs! Everything was falling into place. The integration of our three, often disassociated, selves is the key to living our dreams – the Universe had been trying to tell me that I needed to pull up my anchor all that time ago, but I hadn't been ready to comprehend it back then. Now it was time for me to sail off towards fulfilling my dreams. I felt a surge of happy energy, and I knew that even my Basic Self was beginning to believe it was possible.

My relationship with my parents was continuing to blossom, and it filled me with joy and relief to see them becoming closer again as they were able to enjoy their retirement together. During one weekend trip "home", it dawned on me that the more I had managed to integrate my own, previously disjointed selves, the less snappy and irritable I was with them, which in turn allowed them to reflect more on their own emotions. We were now, for the first time since I was born, able to safely and openly discuss the events of mum's suicide attempts and the impact it'd had on us all. We were able to offer support to each other, and I was so grateful to them for being so supportive of my wish to write about our experiences – it wasn't easy, but we all knew how important it was that stories were heard. Through my own experiences, and subsequent healing, I was able to gradually help mum to see that she didn't need to feel guilty about her own actions, as the consequences had been completely unintentional. I said that, in a funny way, I was actually grateful to her for what she had gone through, as I believed that it had all led me to do what I was doing. We exchanged the same "knowing" look that she and my Nan used to exchange, and could instantly feel the bond between us grow.

"I can't believe it", Mum almost sang to me one day, "I can walk down the street with my head held high, and I can feel things – hunger and excitement – that I've not been able to feel in years; it's like I've been reborn!"

I knew exactly what she meant. Through openly discussing what was behind my mum's distress, and through providing her with peer support, she was now able to finally enjoy the life that she had been prevented from enjoying by her misdiagnosis and consequent heavy medication years ago. *This is what services should consist of,* I allowed myself to daydream about changing the conceptual framework of psychiatry, *a safe place to allow people to openly talk about their own perception of the cause of their emotional distress, in the presence of people who have been through similar experiences, and are able to fully empathise. Maybe that dream would become a reality one day...*

The only way huge societal shifts and policy changes have been made historically has been through people being outspoken about injustice and challenging convention. I needed to be outspoken about the need for change within the mental health system, which I had seen through the transformation of my own mother. My Basic Self may have questioned *who on earth was I to know about changing conceptual frameworks within psychiatry?* but now it had shifted to believing that I was as reputable as anyone else in being part of influencing such a societal shift. I had found the belief within, but I knew that, without conventional qualifications to allow me the power to be recognised, it would be impossible to get my voice heard at a governmental level. One particular psychiatrist, with whom I had the pleasure of coming into contact through a friend and colleague in SCN, Mirabai Swingler, (a fabulous hospital chaplain in South East London), was Dr Russell Razzaque. Mirabai had mentioned Russell the previous year as being one of the few, invaluable, doctors who was open to the ethos of SCN, and I contacted Russell about the impending launch for his book; *Breaking Down is Waking Up.* I told Russell about my own experience and vision for a new, more open-minded mental healthcare service. We became *Facebook* friends and Russell could see how passionate I was about spreading the message – the exact same message he was hoping to spread – that an evolution in psychiatry was desperately needed. We agreed to meet at Alternatives in London to talk before his book launch presentation. On one level it felt surreal; a well-respected and influential consultant psychiatrist was not only taking what I was saying seriously, he was also taking time out of his own schedule to meet me. My energy knew no bounds. On a soul level I knew it was all happening as it was meant to, *the message I channelled **was** actually real.*

EIGHTEEN

WHATEVER NEXT?
A COMPASSIONATE REVOLUTION!

"The secret of change is to focus all of your energy,
not on fighting the old, but on building the new."

SOCRATES

Russell and I sat together in a tiny room below the ground floor of a church in central London. *This is so bizarre!* I laughed inwardly, at one point this situation would have petrified me, but now I couldn't have wished to be anywhere else. We discussed the consequence of living in a scientific era, due to our need for "proof", which has set humankind apart from the natural world – it confines us to the physical Universe and creates a false sense of security related to materialism, which ultimately creates stress, as nothing material can provide stability. Through our shared experiences, Russell and I both knew that stability must first come from within, we both knew that the world view we were trying to change was having a negative impact upon the mental health of the nation as it stood – the mental health of many nations in fact. We had both reached the same conclusion, independently, and from virtually opposite ends of the experiential spectrum; that it was impossible to challenge the current system without having an alternative, proven and improved alternative, to present. We both knew that Socrates was right; it was pointless wasting energy on fighting what was already there, the only option was to get on and prove the need for a new paradigm within psychiatry. I told Russell what had worked with Mum, and what a profound difference it had made to not just her, but everyone connected to her; openly discussing the root of our mutual distress, and me providing empathy and understanding from a peer perspective. And then Russell informed me that he had mooted the idea for an innovative new research study to the medical directors of his Trust, involving merged therapies; Open Dialogue originating from Finland, and Intentional Peer Support originating from New York. He was calling it the POD service – Peer supported Open Dialogue. *Well, this must be exactly what the Universe intends to happen!* we both thought simultaneously.

Acknowledging the need for a paradigm shift within psychiatry doesn't necessitate the need to have had your own spiritual experience, it just necessitates acknowledgement that some people do, and that they need to be given a "safe space" to go through the process and make sense of it in their own way, with non-judgemental support. Having a more open-minded, accepting conceptual framework for psychiatry would, I believe, lead to less prevalence for the need to pathologise what is mostly natural emotional expression to repressed trauma, and consequently reduce the prevalence of said emotional distress. It really isn't rocket-science. I actually find it quite offensive when someone considers my spiritual experiences to be a bit "out-there", because to me they are my normality and completely natural. Open-mindedness in Western society is vital if someone who does encounter "sixth sense" experiences is going to be allowed to be totally self-accepting. And we know through research how vital self-acceptance is to the smooth-running of society as a whole. Internal chaos creates external chaos, and Universal peace can only be achieved if each and every individual finds their own peace inside.

So what do I know about achieving Universal peace? Quite a bit it seems!

The only certain thing is that life is ever changing and flowing, nothing is constant and science doesn't know everything yet – so why do we make assumptions based only on what has been proven so far? This reductionist world view is destroying lives and causing mass mental disease. To live a spiritual life just means to let go of control, of "needing to know" everything, and accept "what is" – this in itself lessens stress. Once we stop fighting ourselves we are free to flourish and grow. Does it really matter what the "truth" is when we can create our own reality with our thoughts anyway? Working to find peace within is not "Hippy shit" as someone had once said to me, it's essential to living a happy and healthy life; there needs to be a paradigm shift in understanding emotion and dealing with it. Transformation is needed not just within psychiatry, but within the education, physical health and prison systems. A shift is happening in science whether we like it or not, so we need to wake up to the new knowledge and make it work for us! I used to think Russell Brand had very strange ideas, but since I woke up I know he speaks the absolute truth and I have the upmost respect for what he has achieved to date.

Nobody has all of the answers. It is by having a democratic alliance of positive activists that together a new paradigm, not only for psychiatry, but for society as a whole, will be able to evolve. Together with Isabel, Dr Bragdon (and lots of valued others), Dr Razzaque and I envisage a coalition of individuals and organisations united in a shared vision to make the mental healthcare system more progressive, hope-inspiring, open-minded and person-centred. The New Paradigm Alliance. It is time to drop our defences and acknowledge that together, with people of all faiths, cultural backgrounds and invaluable experiential knowledge, it is more likely that we will have the answers to achieve more positive outcomes than the current antiquated bio-medical, heavily pharmaceutical-reliant system does. We need to start by having a frank Open-Dialogue amongst ourselves, without hiding behind labels of any kind; professional or patient. It is time to acknowledge that we are all equals, take responsibility, and learn from each other.

It is very fitting that I have received an email with the final version of Isabel's chapter; "Narratives of transformation in psychosis", for the Royal College of Psychiatrists' publication, due at the end of the year. Part of that chapter will be my own written account of my personal transformative journey;

I grew up with a skewed subconscious belief that I was only worthy of living if I was of help to others because my mum had attempted suicide when I was born, and then again when I was seventeen. I felt somehow responsible and as soon as I was old enough, I threw myself into mainstream psychiatry to protect myself with knowledge to prevent "madness" happening to me. The more I learned, the more confused I became, as what I was learning about didn't feel authentic with my soul. Battling to understand resulted in years of feeling inadequate, depressed, and a heavy sense that in order to fit in with a reductionist approach, I had to pretend to be someone I was not.

Holding a "professional" diagnostic view of psychosis and having witnessed my mother being sectioned and given electroconvulsive treatment (she had claimed to be spirit possessed, believing herself to be a "healer") I was petrified that the same would happen to me. My mum had been diagnosed with schizoaffective disorder and was now suffering badly from the side effects of medication.

In 2008 I could no longer maintain my façade of being "okay" and experienced my own mental breakdown. Various traumatic life events took their toll on my already fragile sense of self and I made a serious attempt on my own life. Nothing made sense and living seemed futile. Petrified, knowing I was following in my mother's footsteps, I avoided seeking help, knowing where that would lead. I worked in mental healthcare yet I could not trust the system to provide the support I so desperately needed; it made me feel like a hypocrite.

Then, in March 2012 my belief system about mental illness, the world and my place in it changed literally overnight. During a meditation I experienced a profound breakthrough; the awareness being a soul, I awoke from a state of merely existing as someone who had a mountain of self-doubt to a sense of knowing that I could be anyone I wanted to be. I could reclaim the control of my life I had been longing for but which before that moment I never believed I could have. An absolute sense of pure peace washed over me and I felt that I was totally connected to everything and everyone in the world. I had no sense of anger or fear; everything was taken over by clarity of perspective, acceptance and understanding. At that moment every piece of the jigsaw of my life made complete sense and I had not one regret, I just knew that every crisis had happened to bring me to this moment of strength. My mind had been blessed with a glimpse of another level of consciousness and it would never be the same again. My soul knew that I'd had access to the Universal consciousness, and at this time could freely communicate with spirit. It was an ineffable, amazing experience.

The irony was that having worked within the

mental health system for over twelve years, my educated "logical" brain told me I was psychotic and having delusions of grandiosity. My energy levels at the time were unbounded, and I also feared that I was manic. This chasm of comprehension between my soul and my mind threw me into panic and confusion. Continuing my "normal" daily life without speaking about what I was experiencing at a deeper level was a real challenge, but I feared that if I told anyone who I worked with about my experience, I might end up being hospitalised.

At the same time I suddenly realised that my mum too had been experiencing a spiritual awakening, but not understanding it. The resulting cycle of crisis was aided by myself through my part in getting her sectioned, unable to understand her behaviour at the time. She had spoken about getting "messages" from spirit and being able to predict the future, and I had brushed this off as mad ramblings. Now I recognized our experiences as similar.

Over the last two years I have spoken openly to Mum about spirituality, and acknowledged her own interpretation of her experiences. After more than thirty years of living in an emotionally frozen state, this different narrative has been the only thing that is gradually helping to bring Mum back on the road to recovery. She is no longer locked into a negative belief pattern that she is crazy and worthless. There have been no other changes to her treatment, and the difference in her is astonishing.

Now my mum and I very much see facing the pain as an intrinsic part of our evolutionary process. I consider myself to be hugely lucky. Despite my doubting logical brain, I had the strength of character to listen to my soul, which led me to find a network of people in the UK Spiritual Crisis Network who understood the phenomena of spiritual emergence. With the stability of this conceptual framework to make sense of my experiences and allow natural evolution and integration, it was like coming home – the opposite of seeing psychosis as a destructive illness. I am now more able to be a "silent witness" to my emotions, rather than letting them control me, and I have a much more positive belief system. I know that I am on a life-long journey of learning, but it is now one I enjoy and appreciate.

This positive frame of reference in which to make sense of my experience has both helped me and given me the belief that I can make a positive difference to others. I am now working in collaboration with my local NHS Trust on their spirituality strategy, and am able to provide valuable insight into this different perspective. I am writing a memoir to inspire hope in others who may be suffering. My ultimate mission is to help transform the mental health system in the UK into one that is more positive, progressive and open-minded.

At the moment, the wonderfully positive energies I experience as an acknowledgement that I am on the right path are pretty constant. Being "in the flow" is like living as though Heaven is on Earth. Tears of joy are a regular occurrence, but rather than feeling embarrassed or apologising for expressing my emotions, I welcome them and let them flow; I am only human after all. A normal, emotional human "Being".

As I write this I have synchronistically received an email from Russell.

It contains his confidential draft regarding the objectives and proposed service delivery for the POD. I feel so honoured to be privy to such exciting developments that, ironically, none of the doctors I used to work with (and, in the presence of whom, I felt so inferior) know about. This research study will potentially transform NICE (National Institute for Clinical Excellence) guidelines and policies within the UK, and possibly beyond. It will help to formulate a political transformation agenda to transform how the service that disempowered my mum operates in the future. The Universe has an evolutionary plan, and it is only due to listening to my intuition that I am now in a position to be involved at the heart of it.

Sometimes I celebrate my stubborn streak!

There are times when my Basic Self tries to butt in and make me doubt myself and my abilities; but I am now conscious enough to recognise that I don't need to be controlled by it anymore – I no longer wish to bob around in the harbour, going around in self-doubting circles – it is time to set sail!

There is a need for a radical change in the manner, in which services operate within psychiatry. It is time to acknowledge that we are all on a journey of self-discovery; a journey to Mend the Gap within, in order to Mend the Gap without. We need a service that focuses not on the question;

"What is *wrong* with you?" but instead on the question;

"What *happened to you* to create such an extreme emotional reaction?"

Unlocking the reason behind the trauma empowers the sufferer as they hold the key to the resolution. As a worker, I used to think that my training and knowledge gained from years working in the system meant that I had the answers to help me to help my clients. It wasn't until I had my own breakdown that I realised that the only answers are contained "within the trauma". I am now immensely grateful for my trauma, because without it I wouldn't have had the insight, and the opportunities to self-heal at such a deep level.

The Universe helped me to Mend the Gap within myself, and now it is time to pass on the message it gave me in order to help create that much needed bridge between spiritual experience and psychiatry – The Universe knows it is time to Mend the Gap on a much larger scale;

*I am **just** a vehicle to bring about spiritual awareness; I will help to develop an easily comprehensible framework* *about spiritual crisis to reduce the stigma of mental illness and to increase the understanding of us as spiritual beings within modern society. Mental illness will be redefined in terms of spirituality.*

I know that there is still much for me to learn, but I no longer focus on what I can't do, but instead on what I **can** do, as I know that focus brings me much more positive outcomes. I hope that in some way I have inspired you to do the same. There is however one thing that I will continue to celebrate being bad at for the rest of my life; and that is trying to kill myself. There will always be paradoxes of life to be experienced, and lessons to be learned until the day we die. Whilst writing this book in determination to spread the message, I am working as a Personal Assistant for a lady with Fibromyalgia; she specifically wanted someone to work with her who had spiritual beliefs so that she could be true to herself. It turns out that her emotional sensitivity and clairvoyant abilities had also been misdiagnosed as mental illness in the past. Nothing surprises me anymore. Furthermore, her teenage son has been diagnosed with ADHD. I do not believe he has a "disorder"; he is an empath, extremely sensitive to energies and is also clearly spiritually gifted. He wants to be a platform medium when he's older, and I honestly believe he will do just that. But for now, he is frozen in silence about this natural part of himself when he is outside his home, in fear of being perceived as weird or mental. The problem is that fear could send him mad unless our culture openly acknowledges his truth.

As I am on my knees scrubbing her kitchen floor to make ends meet I realise that, *I may not own much in a material sense any more, but none of that matters because I really **am** living the dream...*

"So whatever turmoil or turbulence life presents to you, know that it has happened for a reason; you broke down so that you may wake up. You got lost so that you may find yourself again."

DR RUSSELL RAZZAQUE,

BREAKING DOWN IS WAKING UP

ACKNOWLEDGEMENTS

I am grateful to the Universe every day for being alive; I now know how truly precious it is to be alive and I try to remember to celebrate it daily.

There are so many people, to whom I am grateful; too many to mention individually here. I am grateful to all of the many wonderful clients (for want of a better word) with whom I have worked over the years, who have been brave enough to share their raw souls with me, which has ultimately led to me being brave enough to expose my own. You taught me so much, and have my upmost respect and gratitude.

I am grateful to the person who saved my life and set me on my spiritual path, without whom I may not be here today, able to relish every sunrise and sunset.

I am grateful to the many wonderful colleagues, with whom I have worked over the years, who were all doing the best they could in a system that was, at times, not only unsupportive of the clients, but also of the staff.

I am particularly grateful to the ones who believed in me, when I didn't believe in myself, some of whom have been mentioned in this book.

I cannot extend enough gratitude to all of the wonderful people involved in the UK *Spiritual Crisis Network*, whose existence saved me from turning my experience into another crisis. I will always be grateful to Catherine Lucas for being brave enough to step outside the box and found the network due to her own experiences.

To the many authors and spiritual teachers who have written about the phenomenon of spiritual awakening, whose books gave me valuable insight and hope when I needed it most; you have all played a part in my transformation.

A special thanks to my fellow "Unleash my spirit" group members; for sitting with me at the beginning of my journey, and taking my (seemingly bizarre) visions seriously. Without your unwavering support and connection, I would not be doing this now! Especially to Linda, who set up the group, and with whom I have shared a very special spiritual journey over the last couple of years; I couldn't have done it without your support soul sister! And Chris, my "Angel Lady" friend, who consistently assured me I wasn't going mad at a time when I feared I was.

Today I am hugely grateful to the brave professionals who are daring to put their head above the parapet and say that changes need to be made within psychiatry. It is a very frightening thing to do, even more so if your professional reputation is at stake. I am grateful to those same professionals for hearing my voice, accepting that it is authentic and worthy of being heard. We are united in a shared mission. I particularly want to thank Professor Chris Cook, Isabel Clarke, Dr Russell Razzaque and Dr Emma Bragdon for all their tireless efforts to make a difference.

Thank you to everyone who made a contribution to *Mend the Gap*, in the form of a personal statement, which can be seen in Chapter 16; you have all helped to give my message more credibility and I am truly honoured.

And finally I am grateful to my parents, for their support and own bravery in enabling me to undertake this project. I understand how difficult it is to feel exposed, and to worry about what people will think. Ultimately we know that it doesn't matter what people think, because we know that going through this process has brought us all much closer to recovery, and if it can help others who may be in similar circumstances, then that is all that matters.

THE AUTHOR

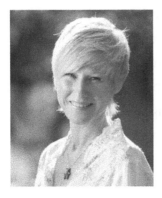 Katie grew up with her mum having been pathologised by the Psychiatric system since experiencing post-natal depression after her birth. This led Katie to want to gain a better understanding of mental illness and she consequently worked within the Psychiatric system for fifteen years. In early 2012, after a period of intense personal crisis, Katie experienced a spiritual awakening, which shook all of the foundations of her conventional learning. This has presented a dichotomy for maintaining a foot in both the psychiatric and spiritual worlds. She hopes that by providing education and support that these worlds will become more harmonious in the future, which will help to alleviate the mental distress experienced by so many in society today.

Katie is a member of the UK Spiritual Crisis Network development group, runs personal and spiritual development workshops, and is involved in the development of an innovative new mental health service, both locally and nationally. Her mission is to normalise the spiritual experience within mainstream society so that spiritual crisis can be more widely acknowledged and supported within mental health services.

Lightning Source UK Ltd.
Milton Keynes UK
UKHW05f1527020818
326661UK00009B/240/P